Vegan, body shaping renaissanc

By Peter Rogers MD.   Copyright February 2021.

"In middle age, I found myself in a dark wood, and the path was lost."
- Dante from "the Divine Comedy."

The Seven deadly dietary sins of health hell

1. ## <u>SATurated fat is SATanic fat</u>. Suicide fat.

   Sat fat reverses mitochondrial electron transport (because beta oxidation excess FADH2), & generates ROS (reactive oxygen species). Mitochondrial failure causes <u>**INSULIN RESISTANCE**</u>, & diabetes. Sat fat elevates **LDL cholesterol**. LDL overcomes RBC zeta potential (negative charge of sialic acid glycocalyx), & causes RBC **rouleaux,** which can last **for 10 hours after one meal**, which increases blood viscosity, & leads to **HTN**, atherosclerosis, & tissue **hypoxia**. Insulin resistance causes **hyperglycemia**, which causes **AGE's** like hemoglobin A1c. AGE's bind R-AGE to activate NADPH oxidase which generates ROS, causing more **oxidative stress**. Hyperglycemia leads to **diabetic** retinopathy, nephropathy, & neuropathy. XS insulin is anabolic, & might function as a tumor promoter. XS insulin depletes insulin-lysin, which appears to limit clearance of beta amyloid, and thus increase risk of Alzheimer's disease (type 3 diabetes). Higher sat fat intake = higher risk of obesity, HTN, diabetes, & Alzheimer's. Brownlee's 2004 Banting lecture is best summary. Sat fat eaters like PIMA have high risk obesity, HTN, MI, DM. Low fat vegetarians opposite. Eg. Tarahumara, Tsimane, Yanomamo, rural Chinese, rural Kenyans, Japanese-Okinawans on rice or on SAD diet. Norwegians, English, Finns & 7d Advents without, or with plants.

2. ## <u>Fructose is F cktose.</u> Drinking fructose (**Frc**) is

drinking "fat." Tons of Frc is put into soda pop, & energy drinks. One 12 oz can contains 50 grams of sugar, & no fiber. ALL Frc goes to your liver as a bolus, & most is converted to fat, as in **FATTY LIVER** = increased obesity, diabetes, serum **ferritin**, ROS, cognitive decline. Blood cholesterol is increased along with risk of atherosclerosis. Frc ain't like glucose. Frc induced fatty liver can progress to cirrhosis. Frc **BYPASSES** the **regulatory** steps in glycolysis. Increased urate is associated with decreased endothelial nitric oxide & increased HTN & gout. **Frc increases Na+ absorption** in gut, and reabsorption by kidneys which worsens HTN. Frc in fruits is different, because contain less Frc (about 4 g per fruit), & more fiber & vitamin C. Fruits are very good for you.

3. ## **Animal protein is a tumor promoter,**

The worst tumor promoter on the planet. The whoore of Babylon attracts you with her makeup (frying, steak sauce, ketchup, salt); unlike a bowl of fruit which all by itself makes you salivate. Teach a man to avoid fish, and you make him healthy for life. TC Campbell noted a dramatic increase in cancer proliferation when dietary animal protein was **10% or higher**. Everybody has some DNA mutated cells, but these only become clinically relevant cancer if promoted. Animal protein increases **ILGF**, a tumor promoter. Meat increases **estrogen** reabsorption in gut, & estrogen stimulates cell proliferation in breast, uterus, & prostate. XS estrogen is a tumor promoter. Meat is high in **methionine** – essential amino acid, for cancer. Meat also high in cysteine. Sulfur from methionine and cysteine gets converted to sulfuric acid, causing **metabolic acidosis**, which is buffered with calcium from bones, leading to osteoporosis & calciuria, with renal tubule precipitation, causing kidney stones, and kidney failure. **Acidotic milieu** favors cancer. High methionine is associated with higher homocysteine, and risk of vascular occlusion. **Leucine** is a branched chain amino acid that stimulates **mTOR** to increase cell proliferation. MTOR is a nutrient sensing system that promotes growth, when nutrients, like leucine, are widely available. Cancer patients do NOT want cell proliferation! Animal protein increases blood cholesterol (that's not a misprint). It's not the cholesterol in the food, it's the food's effect on cholesterol. Animal protein is strongly associated with premature death, which is not surprising given that it is associated with MI, CVA, cancer, & kidney failure. Typical sick person tries to eat more animal protein, and *good* fats. That's why they NEVER get better.

I've seen thousands of patients like this who say, "Well, that's what happens when you get older. It must be genetics. Everyone in my family is fat and sick." When one realizes that health is mostly due to diet, they are empowered to CHANGE what they eat.

4. **Sodium is the silent killer, the snake in the grass**. Na+ inhibits endothelial nitric oxide causing

vasoconstriction & HTN. 75% of dietary salt comes from processed foods. Salted meat causes HTN. Perhaps a new medication could be designed for treatment of hypotension combining the effects of SALt and MEat; call it SALoME. HTN is atherosclerosis risk factor numero uno! Atherosclerosis causes impotence, MI, and stroke. Hunter GATHERERS who eat original diets, like Yanomamo in South America, with very low Na+, about 200 mg a day, don't get hypertension. They can't get no hypertension. Yanomamo don't got no presion alto. None, nada, ninguno. "Low salt" diets that allow 2,000 mg Na+ per day are 10x higher than Yanomamo! Typical box of breakfast cereal has over 2,000 mg Na+, often over 3,000 mg! You will read that the average SAD diet has 3,400 mg Na+/day, but in reality, it's a lot more than that. Walter Kemper limited Na+ to 150 mg/d with great results. Excess dietary Na+ increases calcium loss in urine, and risk of kidney stones, and kidney failure. Healthy humans developed with a low Na+, high K+ diet. Now that's flipped, and they're sick.

5. **PUFA's are the grim reaper of foods.**

Eat PUFA's & you health goes POOF! PUFA's

(PolyUnsaturated Fatty Acids) are not food. Oil is highly processed, liquid fat. Oils are the main reason that philosophic vegans are sometimes fat. Health vegans are always skinny, because they avoid avocados, oils, nuts, and seeds. Omega 6 **PUFA's** contain a "methylene bridge" carbon that's highly vulnerable to lipid peroxidation. **LIPID PEROXIDATION** can initiate chain reactions, like a stack of dominos, that destroy mitochondrial membranes. PUFA's increase risk of macular degeneration blindness, and also inflammation from the arachidonic acid pathway. Mitochondrial dysfunction can lead to cancer. PUFA's predispose to **FERROPTOSIS**. Omega 3's are the fallen angel; not as bad as omega 6, but the halo is gone. All oils are atherogenic; ie. bad for blood flow. Plantiflex Maximus, leader of Vegan church has put

3

PUFA's on the list of forbidden foods.

6. **MSG & aspartame are excitotoxins**,

also known as neurotoxins, and minor "demons." **M**ono**S**odium **G**lutamate, the flavorant, addicts you to junk; like cerebrus, it blocks your exit from health hell. Normal glutamate is L-glutamate. MSG additives contain D-glutamate. Postprandial L-glutamate is sequestered in splanchnic cells to prevent high blood levels of glutamate, which could be neurotoxic. It appears that D-glutamate can partially bypass this regulation. Circumventricular organs, around the brain's third ventricle, lack a blood brain barrier (BBB). Young children BBB's are not fully formed. Old people often have compromised BBB due to diabetes & ischemia. Lack of BBB causes increased vulnerability to MSG. MSG is added to foods under multiple names like "natural flavors," "malt extract," etc.

7. **Excess iron.** Meat is main dietary source of iron (Fe).

Meat Fe is "heme-Fe," which is absorbed much more than plant Fe. Many "multivitamins" & fortified foods contain Fe. The body stores some Fe, so if you get scratched by a tiger, & bleed, you can quickly remake hemoglobin. As Alice Cooper said, "only women [of reproductive age] bleed." The rest of us are high risk to become Fe overloaded. Menstruation is a "therapeutic phlebotomy" that protects women from atherosclerosis. Early age, < 35 yo, **hysterectomy** increases risk of CVA, CHF, & premature **DEMENTIA**! Fe is a transitional metal = variable valence = great for handing off electrons in a controlled setting. Normally, Fe is liganded onto Hb, or enzymes. Unliganded Fe is an oxidant! XS Fe can break free into blood plasma or cell cytoplasm, & become autocatalytic with Fenton chemistry, producing OOdles of reactive oxygen species (ROS). Brent Stockwell showed these ROS can initiate lipid peroxidation chain reactions, & cause ferroptosis (Fe induced ROS causing cell death by lipid peroxidation). Douglas Kell's lab showed that blood has dormant bacteria, essentially "hibernating." We sequester Fe, to prevent reactivation of dormant bacteria, & to prevent other infections. Excess, free Fe in blood can induce a hypercoaguable reaction with fibrinogen, that can accelerate progression of Alzheimer disease, and loss of brain tissue. Increased heme Fe intake (meat) associated with increased diabetes. Meaty, sweety, junk food eat"ee" got more leaky gut"ee" and gums, increasing risk of gut inflammation by LPS (LipoPOlySaccharide from bacterial cell walls), and autoimmune disease like MS, RA, Hashimoto's, via molecular mimicry, and antibody cross reactivity.

Welcome to Health Purgatory:

Restore hope all ye who enter.

Transition time for gut is fast,
A week or two of farts and gas,
That soon will pass.
Then everybody notices,
How slim your waist.
How tight your azz.

You can make it to Health Paradise.

Theme song:

Winners eat starch and fruits,
for six pack abs,
and a horn that toots.

Thesis:

Become a vegan or you're f_cked for health.

Low fat, low salt, whole food, plant eaters are healthier, because that is what we are made to eat; premium fuel for premium performance, mental, physical, and emotional.

Motto:

Vegan today. Vegan tomorrow. Vegan forever!!

Dedication:

To my dear wife Effy. Eff you I love. You are the mother effer of our children. Sometimes I do wish you would eff off.

Contents

Chapter 1

Preface

Why another book?

New stuff learned.

Like what?

Animal protein **accelerates aging** by speeding up arrival of Hayflick limit.

Milk problems are largely synonymous with **FEMALE PROBLEMS**: premature puberty, cramps, PMS, endometriosis, anovulation, breast cancer, ovarian cancer, osteoporosis.

Hysterectomy before age 35, causes increases risk of **DEMENTIA.**

Prostate = uterus = breast.

- Estrogen stimulates proliferation of cells in the prostate, uterus, and breast.

- BPH = fibroids = fibrocystic disease of breast.

- TURP = D&C = lumpectomy for benign breast disease.

- Prostate cancer = endometrial cancer = breast cancer.

- Prostatectomy = hysterectomy = mastectomy.

Prostatectomy causes increased *wish* for dementia.

There is still some magic in that old hat of vitamin C.

The main causes of blindness "C-DAHG" - **C**ataract, **D**iabetes, **A**ging macular degeneration, **H**ypertension, **G**laucoma — are all the same thing = atherosclerosis variants.
The nuance of vitamin **B12**.

And lots more!

Why the jokes about religion and marriage?

People don't care if you make fun of their religion or spouse.

They get offended if you criticize their food choices.

Shakespeare's plays had vulgar jokes for the groundlings, and metaphysical speculations for the learned; ditto for this book.

In the garden, there is a tree of nutrition knowledge of good and evil.

Learn and **live**; ignore and **die**.

The writing is on the wall:

Meat is for chumps.

Vegan is for champs.

Let the Vegan Renaissance begin!

It's up to you to save your soul, but this book will save your ass.

Vegan diet is the most powerful health improver in the world.

Go ahead, read all you want. Your won't find anything more powerful in health science.

I've read the standard medical, nutritional and epidemiological books for the past 30 years.
I've trained with the best doctors, with the best equipment, at the best

8

universities.

Modern medicine helps many people, but vegan diet is the best way to treat obesity, and high cholesterol.

Holy Berry,

Mother of Starch,

Blessed is the fruit of thy womb, Veegus.

Pray for us dietary sinners,

Now and at the hour of our dinners.

What's with the references to paintings?

Hopefully, the occasional metaphors to paintings will make the book more interesting.

During the Italian renaissance, narrative, mural paintings — acres of frescoes —were as common as comic books. Paintings educated the peasants.

In those days, the ignorant masses bought indulgences to try to save themselves. Nowadays, they buy "supplements" to try to make up for their dietary sins.

The art committee assisting with this publication uses elevated standards to select paintings.

The test for skill in female figure drawing is whether a twenty year old virgin male gets aroused by it.

I have to put jokes and art allusions into the book, just to get any readers. I'm more hard up for readers, than Jane Austen was for a husband.

As it is, nobody reads these books. If it were pure biochemistry, then not even nobody would read it.

"Religion is the metaphysics of the masses.

Religion is truth expressed in allegory and myth;

and thus made accessible, and digestible to mankind at large;

for mankind at large could never endure it pure and unalloyed.

Philosophy, on the other hand, should be like the Eleusian Mysteries, reserved for the few and select."

- Arthur Schopenhauer.

Isn't that unscientific?

Most so called "scientific" books gotta lotta nonsense. I've read them.

Biochemistry books recommend high fat diets — that's like recommending cigarettes.

Pathology books say, "NO ONE knows the cause of hypertension," — double digit dummies know that meaty, sweety, salty causes hypertension.

Radiology books say OPLL is a rare disease — every neuroradiologist (if they look for it) sees it every day in atherosclerotic people.

Cardiology books say atherosclerosis is an "inflammatory disease," — then why does it start at bifurcations? Eccentric with clean perivascular margins on CT? Get worse with elevated cortisol?

An inflammatory disease is expected to be diffuse, circumferential, with poorly defined margins = wide transitional zone, rapidly changing, improve with anti-inflammatory cortisol.

I prefer impious truth any day, over "scientific" nonsense. Like Pious Aeneas we shall build a new city of nutrition science.[1]

Why are people so sick?

It's the food!

---

1   **Aeneas**, descendant of Venus (Aphrodite) and Anchises, was the founder of Rome.

Processed food is a powerful poison.

Meat is a moderate poison.

Fructose is liquid fat. Soda pop is bottled fatty liver.

Oils are lubricants for mechanical devices, and perhaps master bay shun, but you shouldn't be eating them. Oils are not food!

The risk factors for atherosclerosis are about the same as the risk factors for cancer.

Meat, oils, fructose, salt, MSG, and estrogenics are OBESOGENS.

Obesity leads to diabetes, impotence, and dementia.

Therefore, these "foods" are also diabetogens, impotogens, and dementogens; **ACCELERANTS OF AGING**.

The average fatso thinks that fish, chicken, and egg whites, are good for them. They love these foods.

They are addicted to the foods that make them sick. That's why they NEVER get better.

It's like mice with **Toxoplasmosis** brain parasites who think that cat piss smells good.

The average middle age man is worried about where he's gonna get his protein; when it's the high protein foods that make him sick.

His **real deficiency is a lack of fiber.** Lack of fiber correlates with increased abdominal pressure syndrome, cancer, and autoimmune disease.

The doctor — who knows what's coming — is like Cassandra or Teiresias[2] — tells the patient once, tells them twice — but they don't listen to his advice.

---

2 **Cassandra** the Trojan prophetess (and Agamemnon's squeeze) could see the future, but no one listened. **Teiresias** the Theban prophet tried to help Oedipus, but he didn't listen – only the wise Odysseus listened to Teiresias. Odysseus was a star in both the "Idiot" and the "Oddity."

To know the truth about chronic disease prevention, but have no one listen, is the **vegan man's burden.**

What about the food pyramid that recommends meats and sweets?

That pyramid killed my mummy — she died of colon cancer from eating meat.

That pyramid is a a tower of babble.[3]

Are you recommending a new pyramid?

Yes.

The forever young, forever potent, pyramid has only 4 levels.

#1. B12.	***** B12 *****
#2. Vegetables.	******* Veggies *******
#3. Fruits.	************ Fruits **************
#4. Starch.	*************** Starch *****************

Starch, fruits, and vegetables are THE three food groups; the "Holy Trinity" of foods.

We'll add B12 as a token *female* food to signal our virtue, like Mary who was made Queen of Heaven.

Therefore, Veganism is a pagan religion with at least the 4 gods of starch, fruits, vegetables, and B12.

---

3 **"Tower of Babel"** painted by Pieter Breugel.

Aren't pagans low life scum?

Homer, Aesop, Aeschylus, Sophocles, Euripides, Aristophanes, Socrates, Plato, Aristotle, Thales, Pythagoras, Archimedes, Virgil, Vitruvius, Ovid, Cicero, Quintilian, and Epictetus were pagans.

Catholics pray to saints as if they were gods, so they're pagans.[4]

Italian renaissance humanists combined classic religions with Catholicism so they were pagans.[5] Michelangelo painted the Cumean Sibyl, priestess and prophetess of Apollo, adviser of Aeneas, on the Sistine Chapel ceiling.

"I sing of starches, fruits and the man."   -Virgil.[6]

What about avocados, nuts, and seeds?

Young people can eat them in **small** amounts. The over 40 crowd should avoid them;

except for a couple of times a year during the holidays. Otherwise, got too much fat for people over 40.

Some seeds are high in estrogen.

Fat is bad. Really bad; as this book will show. The only fat you need to eat is the little bit that comes from low fat, plant foods.

Nathan Pritikin was right when he said, "Fat is bad."

"Good fats" and "Mediterranean diet" are Trojan horse slogans to get the gullible to eat meat and oils.

Dorothy was right when she said, "There's no place like home.
There's no place like home."
There's no good fats. There's no good fats.

---

4   **"Apotheosis of St Ignatius"** painted by Andrea Pozzo in 1694. One of the best ceiling murals ever painted.
5   **"School of Athens"** painted by Raphael in 1510.
6   Parody of opening line from "The Aeneid" by Virgil.

What's the most important thing to know about food?

Low fat, low sodium, plant foods make people skinny and healthy.

The best path to health is low fat, low sodium, whole food, 100%, plant based diet with,

STARCH and FRUITS to SATISFY HUNGER,

and vegetables for extra nutrients.

You've gotta satisfy your hunger or you will fall off the wagon.

Even though Dr McDougall is the greatest nutrition expert in the world, and one of my heroes, I think he's wrong about fruits.

He wrote that people should only eat about 10% of their calories from fruits, and about 70% from starch — (and the other 20% from vegetables). He wrote that fruits can have too much simple sugars to be eaten in large amounts.

Yes. Some fruits like bananas do have too much sugar for me.

Some fruits like watermelon and pineapple are packed with sugar, but compensate by diluting it with their high water content.

However, other fruits like wild blueberries (6 grams per serving), have more fiber than oatmeal (4 grams per serving); and less protein, and they're alkaline. Yum, yum, healthy, healthy.

Dr McDougall emphasizes that healthy populations have eaten starch based diets for thousands of years, for all of recorded history.

That's great, but what did they eat before that?

I'll bet a big part of their diet was fruits, and that our metabolic system is designed for more than 10% of our calories from fruit; and our color vision was "given" to us so we could see when a fruit was ripe.
Cyrus Wombatta and Bobby Bigpoo of "Mastering diabetes" fame live as "fruitarians," and they seem quite healthy.

"Fully mature intellects love truth, even when it appears plain and simple, boring to the ordinary person;

for they have noticed that truth tends to reveal its highest wisdom in the guise of simplicity."
- Nietzsche.

What's your prediction for the future of nutrition?

America will have three food castes.

The **lowest caste** — the proles — will eat processed food, fast food, and sugary drinks. The typical meal is burger, fries, and soda. At home, they drink tap water. They will become fat and sick in their thirties with hypertension, diabetes, and heart disease. For health care, proles present late with advanced disease to emergency rooms. They will usually die between 50-65 years old; so a lot of money will be saved for social security.

The **middle caste** — the bourgeoisie — will avoid fast food, but will still eat meat. At home they drink carbon filtered water. They will become fat and sick in their 40's and 50's. They will go to nurse practicioners who type their symptoms into a computer, and then an artificial intelligence program prints out a list of pills, or refers them to surgical specialists. They get all the diseases that require surgery like kidney stones, appendicitis, diverticulitis, cholecystitis, and cataracts. They die around 60-75 years old.

The **highest caste** — the aristocrats — will be 100%, low fat, low sodium, whole food vegans. They are slim and trim, all their lives, and seldom have any health problems. Their biggest problem is figuring out how to get laid that weekend. At home, they drink reverse osmosis water (after eating, but not before, because too low in osmolality). They will maintain their sexual potency into their 80's, and will have orgies in the nursing homes. If they can avoid neurosyphilis, they will often live to be 100.

If you want to become a Queen Bee, you've got to eat royal jelly; junk food ain't gonna do it.

What's the big picture with nutrition and health?

The economy runs on fat people.

Nobody's making money off skinny vegans.

Fat people are cash cows for:

- Corporations (lowered pensions because die soon after retirement).

- Big food (they eat a lot of junk food).

- Divorce industry (get divorced a lot because women have contempt for fat husbands, and men do not want to have sex with fat wives).

- Hospitals (they get TONS of chronic diseases).

- Makers of canes and motorized wheelchairs.

Like the controlled, slow, oxidation of glucose to provide energy for making ATP;

Fat people undergo a controlled, slow removal of their money to provide energy for the economy.

Lambs of god, you take away the sins of the planned economy.

Thank gods for fat people.

What's the elevator pitch for vegan diet?

In 2020, the most common cause of premature death was progression of chronic disease.

The #1 cause of death is myocardial infarction (MI) at 26% of the population.

The incidence of MI in low fat vegans is less than 1% (see Dr Caldwell Esselstyn's paper in 2014, journal of family practice).

The #2 cause of death is cancer at 25%.

Low fat vegans have the lowest risk of cancer.

The more meat you eat, the higher your risk of cancer death.

The 3rd, 4th, 5th, 6th, 7th, most common causes of death — stroke, diabetes, kidney disease, vascular dementia, and Alzheimer's — all cull about 5%.

Low fat vegans have the lowest risk of stroke, diabetes, kidney disease, vascular dementia, and Alzheimer's.

The other killer diseases that also take about 5% can usually be avoided — COPD (don't smoke) — trauma (avoid alcohol).

Most people die prematurely, because they ignorantly poison themselves with bad food, alcohol, tobacco, and estrogenic chemicals.

What's the longest, average life span?

He who controls cholesterol, controls arterial patency; he who controls arterial patency, controls longevity.

The longest average life span, that is well documented, is for the vegan Seventh Day Adventists, in Loma Linda, California, with the women at 89.6 years, and the men at 87 years.

Dr John McDougall worked with that population, and he said that many of the persons in the top category were not as careful with their diet and lifestyle as the study suggests; and he thinks the average lifespan for a truly low fat vegan, who avoids tobacco and alcohol, is actually higher than 87-89.6 years.

Other researchers believe that the Okinawans had a longer average life expectancy than 87-89.6 years, but it's not as well documented.

What's the bottom line for maximal lifespan?

If a population eats low fat, low sodium, whole food vegan, and avoids alcohol, and tobacco, walks every day, and maintains some social connections, they can probably live an average of 95 years.

Why are old people more fragile?

Loss of ascending thoracic aorta elastic fibers, which can't be replaced after 28 years of age, and causes a decrease in Windkessel effect.

Loss of endothelial precursor cells (EPC's), which are stem cells to repair arteries with atherosclerosis.

Accumulated atherosclerosis causing less blood flow to tissues.

Loss of muscle mass, meaning that when they fall, they often fracture their hips, and spines.

Sleep problems. Weaker immune systems.

Trend towards more salt sensitivity for development of hypertension.

The older you get, the more fragile you get; so the more careful you have to be, if you want to stay healthy.

What's the difference between plant and animal foods?

Good stuff comes from plants, like fiber, antioxidants, and carbohydrates.

Bad stuff comes from animals like sat fat, animal protein, and heme.

Animals stabilize cell membranes with cholesterol, so animal foods always contain cholesterol.

Plants stabilize cell membranes with cellulose (fiber), so **plant foods always contain fiber.**

Animal foods have no fiber, and almost zero antioxidants.

Animal foods tend to be stored or flavored with **sodium**, which is a vaso**CONSTRICTOR**, causing hypertension, and atherosclerosis.

Plant foods tend to be high in **potassium** which is the opposite of sodium. Potassium is a vaso**DILATOR**, which lowers blood pressure (BP), and helps prevent atherosclerosis.

Research has shown, that the more sodium humans eat, the higher their BP, for example with the DASH study.

When chimpanzees have sodium added to their diet, their BP goes up. When the sodium is removed, their BP goes down.

Plant foods have lots of antioxidants; that's how plants survive in the hot sun all day.

Plant foods are high in **FOLATE** which helps prevent cancer, by maintaining thymine levels. If folate is deficient, then thymine levels drop, and uracil gets inserted into DNA. Uracil insertion into DNA causes mutations. See chapter on vitamin B12.

Plant foods are high in nutrients, and low in calories. Low caloric density stretches the stomach with fewer calories to provide early satiety.

Fiber slows absorption of glucose from gut to blood, to keep blood glucose normal for a prolonged amount of time, prolonged satiety.

Starch and fruits satisfy hunger with the fewest calories; and therefore optimize bodyweight; and optimize longevity — the HAPPY path to "caloric deprivation."

Low fat, plant foods — which means almost all plant foods, except avocados, nuts, and seeds — are primarily **carbohydrate and fiber**.

Animal foods are low in nutrients, and high in calories. Animal foods are primarily **protein and fat**. It takes thousands of calories to stretch your stomach with animal foods.

A **typical meat is 50% fat and 50% protein**. A recipe for **DEATH**. Run for your life!

Animal protein (leucine, methionine), and animal fat (mostly saturated fat) are bad for you.

The only person who benefits from animal foods is a young weight lifter who wants to gain weight fast, or a refractory epileptic or an IDA anemic.

For everyone else, animal foods do not have any redeeming value.

Show me a middle aged **meat eater**, and I'll show you **plugged up arteries**.

Show me a low fat, low sodium **vegan**, and I'll show you **clean arteries**.

The most important thing for health is good blood supply.

Heads, shoulders, knees, and toes; all work better when blood flows.

"With English Churches, everything Catholic is glorious; everything Protestant is debased."   - AWN Pugin.[7]

With food, everything, whole food, low fat vegan is glorious; everything meaty, sweety, oily is debased.

"All art is either instruction or infection."   - John Ruskin.[8]

All food is either healthy or unhealthy.

"It's the glory of Gothic architecture that it can do anything."
                                                            - John Ruskin.

It's the glory of the low fat, vegan diet, that it can do almost anything;

It's the only diet shown capable of reversing coronary artery disease, and it can often reverse type 2 diabetes and hypertension, and it routinely reverses obesity.

"All things are possible to him that believeth."   - Mark 9:23.

Almost all things are possible to him that eateth the proper diet.

So far it can't raise the dead, but Walter Kempner MD,[9] and Caldwell Esselstyn,[10] saved some persons who were nearly dead.

---

7   AWN Pugin was lead architect in England's Gothic revival in the 1800's.
8   John Ruskin lead art and architecture critic at Oxford in the 1800's.
9   Walter Kempner is the "rice diet" genius of North Carolina.
10   Caldwell Esselstyn is the king of "prevent and reverse heart disease."

How can you tell if a person is a nutrition ignoramus?

They say stupid stuff like:

Everything in moderation.

- Yeah, brilliant. Put good food on half your plate, and junk on the other half.

- Why not put good food on both sides.

I prefer the Mediterranean diet.

- Oh really? Which Mediterranean are you talking about?

- Ancient Greeks were heroic. Modern Greeks are fat.

- Most "Mediterranean" diet types are following a diet from Crete, for Cretins.

I'm trying to cut down on carbs.

- Saying carbs is like saying "hot-cold," or "good-bad."

- As soon as someone says "carbs," an "I'm an idiot" sign appears over their head.

- A nutritionally educated person knows the difference between simple and complex carbohydrates.

I'm a flexitarian.

- Another melodius slogan to excuse eating junk food.

I can eat whatever I want, because I exercise a lot.

- Oh really? Look what happened the mensa, marathon runner, Jim Fixx, who failed his instant IQ test.

- Jim Fixx, "Mr sexy legs," was on top of the world with his running, until he died of an MI at 52 years old. His coronaries were severely atherosclerotic.

- Look what happened to Bob Harper, the world famous, super trainer, who had a massive MI at 52 years of age.

- Sat fat conquered his six pack abs. He was saved by defibrillation.

I love the taste of junk food.

- No sh_t. Chemicals are added to it, to make people addicted to it.

- Your body is a sophisticated, metabolic machine. Eating junk food is like throwing a monkey wrench into the gears.

I didn't used to be fat. This must be a thyroid problem.

- It's reasonable to check a TSH level, but that's seldom the cause.

- What's the best way to reduce risk of autoimmune diseases like Hashimoto's thyroiditis, or Grave's disease?

- Eat a low fat, 100% whole food, vegan diet!

This fatness must be a hormone problem.

- What is the most common cause of elevated estrogen? Eating meat.

- What are common causes of increased estrogen exposure? Aluminum deodorant, cosmetics, BPA laundry detergent, etc.

- This topic is discussed in more detail in the chapter on "female problems."

I don't care about living to be 100, I just want to enjoy my meals.

- The goal is to be as healthy as possible, for as long as possible. Quality matters.

- The MOFU diet (Meat, Oils, Fructose, Unknown additives) diet is not that enjoyable.

- Becoming fat and impotent is not fun. Becoming diabetic, and having to poke yourself with needles everyday to check your blood sugar is not fun.

- Meat eater diseases often need to be surgerized; getting cut open is not fun.

Plant foods are boring?

- Your tastes will change. Plants seem simple at first.

- It's like looking at a renaissance painting. At first it seems plain, perhaps a little flat, Byzantine-ish.

- But when you look at in context, as part of a story, like the *prodigal son;* then it's more appealing.

- On the one hand, it's sad that most Catholics are functional illiterates; on the other hand, efforts to educate them with painting and sculpture, have created a lot of great art.

- That simple plant food provides fiber to feed your good gut bacteria, who feed your colon enterocytes, to prevent leaky gut.

- That fiber slows glucose absorption, so your blood glucose level stays normal, for a prolonged amount of time.

- The starch, fruits, and vegetables work together to create a coordinated, symphony of health.

- It's like seeing that the painting goes in harmony with the tapestries, stained glass windows, and sculptures, and great arches in the Cathedral. And the whole effect resonates, and is beautiful.

- You are the **Prodigal Son**; coming home to join the family of foods where you belong, as a starchivore-frugivore-veggivore.

- Cats are pure carnivores. Dogs are true omnivores. You are meant to be a plantivore.

How can I cook without oil? I need oil for cooking.

- Cooking oils didn't exist before 1880. People somehow managed before then.

- Oils are to human health, what barbarians were to the health of Rome in 476 AD.

- The only thing you need to make rice, oatmeal, quinoa, potatos, sweet potatos, and beans, is to boil water, which can often be done with a pressure cooker.

- Fruits are eaten raw.

- Most vegetables don't need to be cooked.

- There are lots of vegan cookbooks.

How do I cook?

- I cook the old fashioned way. I have women do it.

- My muses don't help me much with writing, but they make a good breakfast.

- Isn't that sexist?

- No. That's what mamas, grandmas and wives want. Contrary to popular legend, women are not that nice. There's no Florence Nightingales in the kitchen.[11]

- You can't avoid the split tails in the kitchen.

- Women are territorial animals, that maintain control of the kitchen by bitching at anyone who goes near the sink.

- You're wasting water! You just splashed the window. Now, clean it up! I'm sick and tired of cleaning up after you! Move! I need to peel potatos!

---

11 **Florence Nightingale** was a nurse who dramatically improved survival rates in English hospitals in the 1800's with better nutrition, sanitation, ventilation, and kindness. She was lovingly nicknamed "the Lady of the Lamp."

- My mother — who was the gentlest woman in the world — told me that if I ever again brushed my teeth, and rinsed my mouth over the kitchen sink — [her territory] — that she was going to kill me.

What about all those people who say that meat is "good for you"?

They are like astrologers.

"How happy are astrologers; to be believed if they tell a truth once out of one hundred lies. When other persons are not believed if they tell one lie."
- Frances Guiciardini, renaissance historian.

Other than increasing your risk of obesity, HTN, diabetes, cancer, infertility, premature death, myocardial infarction, stroke, kidney stones, kidney failure, osteoporosis, diverticulitis, appendicitis, blindness, Alzheimer's disease, autoimmune disease, and impotence, meat is *good* for you.

Is the dietary connection of meat, oils, salt, sugar (MOSS), and disease a new discovery?

In the 1400's the Florentines rediscovered the science and literature of the Greeks and Romans to start the Italian renaissance.

In the 2000's, we are rediscovering the science of the 1900's to usher in the **VEGAN RENAISSANCE**.

Upon reading about Walter Kempner's incredible results with the rice diet in the mid 1900's, I felt like Heinrich Schlieman, unearthing Troy, and finding the "Treasure of Priam."[12]

The research has already been done; we just need to learn about it.

In fact, the best diet for humans has been known for a long time, and it's

---

12 **Priam** was the king of ancientTroy. Heinrich **Schlieman**, the father of archeology, located ancient Troy. He claims to have found the necklace and crown (diadem) from **Helen of Troy**; which he gave to his wife.

called the **"Genesis diet."**

*T*hen God said, "Behold, I have given you every **PLANT** yielding seed, which is upon the face of all the earth, and every tree which has fruit; it shall be food for you.

- Genesis 1:29.

The Bible is the Romulus and Remus of nutrition books.

How can we prove that 100% vegan, low fat, low salt is better?

The obvious answer is look at epidemiology like the Okinawans, Japanese migration studies, Tarahumara, 7th Day Adventists, Yanomamo, Brazilian Xingu, Bolivian Tsimane, Ikarian Grecians, Italian Sardinians, new and improved Finns, Nicoyan Costa Ricans, rural Kenyans, rural Chinese, rationing events in Denmark, Norway, England, Cuba, as well as many other plant based populations.

Botticelli painted *Birth of Venus;* Vegan diet *restores peenus* function in many.[13]

A flaccid peenus is a warning sign that coronary, and carotid atherosclerosis are on the way.

Find a friend with mild impotence, and ask him to go vegan for one month.

Don't be surprised if his Bonnie comes back to life.

Such is the legend of the true diet.[14]

---

13 **"Birth of Venus"** by Botticelli, painted in 1486.
14 **"Recognition of the true cross"** by Piero della Francesca, painted in 1465.

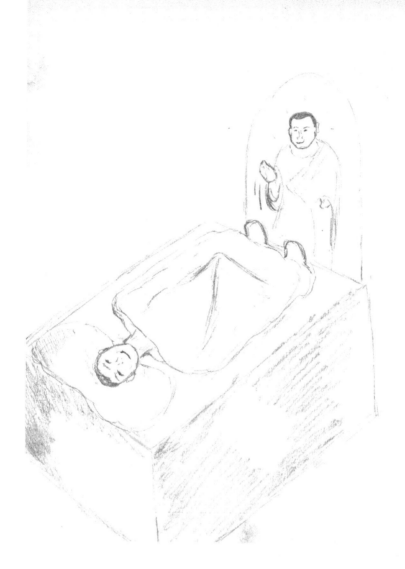

Drawing Caption: Lazarus bon_r come back to life.

What is the prayer for impotence patients?

Padre Nuestro

Our Father who art in boner land,
Solid wood be thy name.

Give us this day our daily boner,

And forgive us our dietary sins,

As we forgive those who misdiet against us.

And lead us not into temptation,

but deliver us from impotence.

What is the Vegan Creed?

We believe in one Diet, the Vegan Diet almighty, the father of all diets,

creator of heaven on earth, maker of thin bodies, and opener of arteries.

We believe in the Vegan Diet, the only diet that optimizes health.

Increaser of nitrous oxide, alkalinizer of blood,

optimizer of immune system, soother of inflammation.

Eternally begotten by mother nature.

Of the same substance as nature.

God from goddess. Sunlight from sunlight.

Vegan diet for us, and for our salvation.   Amen.

What is the Vegan theme song?

Amazing Starch

> Amazing STARCH,
> how sweet the sound
> that saved a SLOB like me.
>
> I once was FAT, but now I'm THIN,
> was blind, but now I see.

Twas STARCH that taught my ARTERIES to FLOW,
And STARCH my blockages relieved.

How precious did that STARCH appear,
the hour I first believed.

What's the best workout music for Vegans?

Veggae and Veggaeton.

You probably know some of the more famous Veggae songs like:

"I shot my wad,

but I didn't come inside her."

Are there any songs for Vegan Saints?

Old McDougall had a farm[15]

Old McDougall had a farm,
V-e-g-a-n.
And on that farm he had some rice,
with some chopsticks here, and some chopsticks there.
V-e-g-a-n.
And on that farm he had some yams.
With a dig, dig here, and a dig, dig there.
V-e-g-a-n.

What movie has the best line to motivate vegans?

Animal house. Dean Wormer told Flounder, "Fat, drunk, and stupid is no way to go through life."

MOFU (Meat, Oils, Fructose, Unknown additives) causes obesity, sickness,

---

15 John McDougall MD is one of the best nutrition doctors in the world.

and cognitive impairment.

Fat, sick, and stupid is no way to go through life.

What other titles were considered for this book?

Most "learn Spanish" books are "intro" to Spanish. Same thing with nutrition and pathophysiology books.

There is a great intermediate to advanced book for learning Spanish called, "Breaking out of beginner Spanish."

This book could be called, "Breaking out of beginner Nutrition and Pathophysiology."

What about constipation?

A constipated butt is a warning sign that abdominal pressure syndrome, and cancer are tailing you.

Normally, you should have **at least** 2 poops a day.

Fiber is the best answer for many abdominal problems.

Normally, you should eat at least 40 grams of fiber per day, ideally around 100 grams per day.

The higher your fiber intake **from whole plant foods**, the lower your risk of obesity, hypertension, diabetes, colon cancer, breast cancer.

I eat an average of 105 grams of fiber per day.

One serving of oat meal has 4 grams of fiber. One apple has 4 grams of fiber. One serving of wild blueberries has 6 grams of fiber.

Where does all this knowledge about fiber, and constipation come from?

Dr Burkitt discussed in the next chapter.

Disclaimer:

Vegetarian diet can cause a drop in blood pressure and blood glucose for people on medications.

You should let your doctor know before beginning a vegetarian diet.

Vegan diet can decrease the need for blood pressure pills.

Vegan diet also can decrease the need for diabetes medications.

Disclosure:

Dr Rogers is an Amish mechanic. He is not a clinical doctor. He's just a radiologist who doesn't even know the dose of aspirin. He does not actually manage the medications or nutrition of any real patients.

He simply provides nutritional information to people who ask, and then they usually ignore him, and never ask again.

The statements in this book are not intended as a substitute for professional medical advice.

This book is for educational purposes only, and should not be used to diagnose or treat any illness.

Dr. Rogers is not your health care provider, and never will be, unless you meet him in person, and that's hard to do, because he's a semi-autistic, hermit recluse.

He does not sell any supplements.

He does not receive financial support from any companies.

Financially, he is kind of a loser.

Chapter 2

Fiber man, Dennis Burkitt

Why are modern people so fat and sick?

        a. Lack of fiber

        b. Excess sugar

        c. Excess fat

        d. Excess oil

        e. All of the above.

Answer: All of the above.

Dr. Denis Burkitt and abdominal pressure syndrome.

Dr Denis Burkitt is the patron "saint" of fiber.

Burkitt was an Irish surgeon, who worked as a Christian missionary doctor in Africa, in the 1950's and 1960's.

Burkitt did his surgery residency in England, where he saw all the typical Meat, Oil, Salt, Sugar (MOSS) diet diseases.

In Africa, he saw two patients with unusual jaw tumors, and he checked around all the other hospitals in Africa, to see if anyone else, had seen this type of tumor.

Burkitt traveled in a jeep — 10,000 miles — throughout Africa to map the occurrence pattern of this jaw tumor.

Cancer causation by viruses was a hot topic in those days, and the research world was eager to see if "Burkitt's" lymphoma was caused by a virus.

The research community was so impressed by Burkitt's tumor mapping, that he was promoted to become a medical epidemiologist — the best job for a nutrition researcher.

Burkitt did not become interested in lack of fiber as a cause of disease, until he was 56 years old!

Peter Cleave MD asked the now famous Burkitt to help him promote his theory that the main cause of chronic diseases — like atherosclerosis, stroke, and cancer — was TOO MUCH SUGAR.

Before 1970, sugar meant "sucrose." Sucrose is a combination of glucose plus fructose. High fructose corn syrup did not become widespread until the 1970's.

Then Hugh Trowell MD asked Burkitt to help him promote his theory that the main cause of chronic disease was LACK OF FIBER.

At the same time, Nathan Pritikin — the genius scientist who saved himself from coronary artery disease — was convinced that the main problem was TOO MUCH FAT, and that ALL FAT WAS BAD.

By the way, they're all right. We'll parse out the details in the next chapters.

History of food and disease:

The industrial era of the 1800's brought with it "modern diseases."

In the 1800's:

Rural people moved to the cities, and inhaled more air pollution.

Railroads and motor cars enabled transport of meat to the cities.

Refined sugar became available, and was added to food.

Refined oils, like cottonseed oil, became available in the 1880's.

Trans fats were added to the diet in 1912.

Before 1920, most premature death was due to infections like cholera, TB, syphilis, and strep throat with rheumatic fever.

In the modern, industrialized world, a kid with a swollen knee means that he got injured playing sports — meniscal tear, or cruciate ligament tear.

My dad, growing up in Ireland in the 1930-40's said that if a kid had a swollen knee, everybody would say, "Oh, must be TB."

Before 1920, you couldn't find myocardial infarction, or macular degeneration in a medical textbook.

By the mid 1900's most premature death in adults was due to myocardial infarction, stroke, and cancer.

By the mid 1900's other "modern" diseases were becoming common like macular degeneration, cataract, glaucoma, gallstones, cardiac angina....

Nowadays, a doctor does not even need to look at the chart, to know that "fat, 60 year old man" is synonymous with hypertensive, diabetic with coronary artery disease, and impotence.

Burkitt saw that Western diets created a **WHOLE NEW PATTERN OF DISEASE**. Diseases that did not happen in persons eating traditional, endemic, plant based diets.

Burkitt concluded that fiber was the most important variable. Meat and refined flour — typical of Western diets — cause a SLOW intestinal transit time, with small, hard stools.

The healthy, African populations he worked with ate mostly **sweet potatos and brown rice**, and had faster intestinal transit time.

How can you test your own bowel transit time?

With beet juice. Beet juice makes your poop red.

Food travels through your small bowel in 3 hours, but it spends 36 hours in your colon.

Red poop two days later is normal.

Red poop four days later means you're constipated.

Why does food stay so long in the colon?

Mostly for water reabsorption, but also for vitamin K absorption, and electrolyte balance.

What about Burkitt and abdominal pressure syndrome?

Burkitt noted that Irish manual laborers were healthy on a daily diet of ten pounds of potatos a day, and a pint of milk.

Are potatos good for you?

Dr John McDougall, the great nutrition doctor, says that potatos and sweet potatos are the best foods in the world because:

- Grow well in harsh conditions.

- Provide a lot of calories per acre.

- Are nutritionally complete; you can live off of potatos and water.

In the 1840's with the potato famine, the English tried to starve the Irish, and largely succeeded, with the Irish population decreasing from 8 million, to 4 million.

Luckily, the descendants of Burkitt and McDougall survived to provide the world with the two best nutrition doctors of the 1900's.

What about abdominal pressure syndrome?

Dr Burkitt also observed that vegetarian persons had bigger stools.

Vegetarians had much less constipation, diverticulitis, appendicitis, hiatal hernia, and gastroesophageal reflux (GERD).

Fiber is only present in plant foods.

In the colon, fiber binds to fluid, so that plant eaters have softer stools.

Appendicitis is caused by dry, hard stool — fecaliths — obstructing the appendix. Appendix glands keep secreting mucus, but the mucus is blocked by the fecalith.

Then the appendix pops, and stool is spilled into the peritoneum (the space around the bowel).

Plant eaters have liquid stool on the right side of the colon, and therefore less appendicitis.

Softer stools means less straining during defecation.

Less straining means less back pressure on the abdomen.

Less back pressure means less diverticulosis (outpouchings on the sigmoid colon), and therefore less diverticulitis (outpouchings that pop, and leak stool into the peritoneum).

Less back pressure also means less hiatal hernia (stomach bulging into the chest), and less GERD (Gastro Esophageal Reflux Disease).

Burkitt named this pattern of diseases "ABDOMINAL PRESSURE SYNDROME."

Abdominal pressure syndrome means that meat diet constipation causes straining at defecation with increased intra-abdominal pressure.

The increased abdominal pressure causes diverticulosis, hiatal hernia, GERD, hemorrhoids, spermatocele, varicocele and **VARICOSE VEINS**.

Women are impressed when you tell them it causes varicose veins.

Men say things like, **"You telling me my balls ache, (spermatocele, varicocele, hernia) because I'm constipated?"**

He found that many persons would approach him years after hearing one of his lectures to tell him that they still remembered his pictorial illustrations.

Consequently he came to believe that a picture was a FAR more valuable teaching tool than words, or even humorous allusions, though his lectures were also full of these.

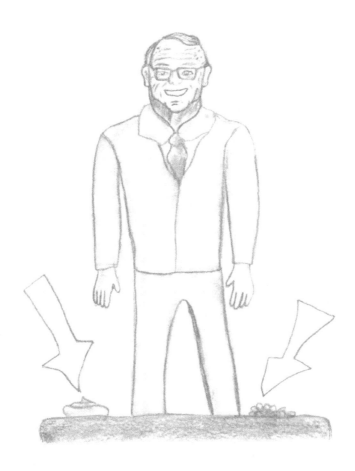

Caption: Dr. Denis Burkitt "pointing" to the big soft stool of a vegan on his right and the hard dry pellets of stool from a meat eater on his left.

The following are quotes of Dr. Denis Burkitt:

"Better to build a fence at the top of the cliff than to park an ambulance at the bottom...

Prevention can eliminate disease, but early diagnosis and good treatment can only rarely eliminate disease...

our bodies are adapted to a stone age diet of roots and vegetables...

if people pass small stools, you need large hospitals...

the **ONLY WAY TO REDUCE DISEASE** is to go backward to the diets and lifestyles of our ancestors...

in twenty years with a [vegetarian population] I only had to remove one gallstone.

The citizens of countries that don't get bowel cancer, don't get bowel polyps either...."
                                                              - Denis Burkitt.

In the chapter on Leaky Gut, the topic of fiber will be discussed in more detail.

Chapter 3

Alzheimer prevention with Notre Dame Nuns and cognitive reserve

If I get reincarnated, I'd like to be in charge of a convent. That would be a great set up for polygamy.

No male competition. Naive women. Just say the kids were adopted. Someone else pays the bills. Perrrrrrfect.

Notre Dame nuns in Mankato, Minnesota donated their brains to science. At death, autopsy was performed, to check for Alzheimer's disease.

Nuns are good for research, because virtually no alcohol, tobacco, Ob-Gyne, or other pesky variables.

The big finding was that the nuns — who were more literary — and academic — were less likely to develop Alzheimers.

Some of the "academic" nuns did have Alzheimer brain lesions — like beta amyloid plaques, and neurofibrillary tangles — but they were **ASYMPTOMATIC**.

Having extra **cognitive reserve** protects against Alzheimer's disease.

It is good to keep your mind stimulated with intellectual activity. Enriched environment can be whatever you enjoy for reading, writing, teaching, and hobbies.

One definition of health is "**VITALITY**." The nuns with more intellectual vitality remained asymptomatic, despite some brain lesions.

Physical vitality is equally important. When a healthy person trips and falls, they put out their hands to absorb the impact, and it's no big deal — more embarrassment than anything else.

When fragile old people fall, they often get brain bleeds, and spine fractures.

In the movie, "It's a wonderful life," Jimmy Stewart's daughter said, "Every time a bell rings, an angel gets her wings."

In the modern world, every time an old guy falls, the emergency room, cash register sings.

Old guy falls — check CT head, cervical spine, thoracic spine — check blood test for anemia — check EKG for arrhythmia etc.

Health is like a video game. Like a video game where you can build up **"energy" points,"** that give you capacity to tolerate injuries; you can build reserve "energy" in physical, emotional, and intellectual ways.

Hans Selye — the great researcher on psychological stress — said that, "Every time we suffer an injury, the penalty we pay for healing, is **accelerated aging**."

Time for a séance.

!#^$@^|💱!☺☼♀🐂♂☁☺☁🐚🙈🙉🙊

The Sibyl of Cumea, priestess of Apollo, is sending a vision, a prophecy for the future: right now the affluent societies are flooded with fat diabetics. Soon this flood will turn into a tsunami of Alzheimer's patients.

Alzheimer's is type 3 diabetes. Insulin degrading enzyme is the same enzyme that removes beta amyloid from the brain. Saturated fat related insulin resistance leads to hyperinsulinemia.

Increased insulin means increased risk of Alzheimer's disease.

Hyperinsulinemia depletes insulin degrading enzyme, which can only be made in limited quantities. Beta amyloid accumulates in the brain. Alzheimer's becomes symptomatic. Grandma and grandpa don't know what day it is.

Take home message:

Build physical reserve with exercise, and low fat, low sodium, whole food, plant based diet.

To maintain health, our rate of repair must be greater than our rate of injury. Healthy habits help us to maintain our DNA repair systems, endothelial precursor stem cells (EPC's), and thoracic aorta elastic fibers (to maintain Windkessel effect).

<u>Build emotional reserve</u> by developing social skills, having a good PURPOSE in life, and studying philosophy like stoicism. Epictetus is a great stoic.

"Inferior people blame others for their problems. [Everybody in my family is fat. It's genetic.]

Ordinary people blame themselves. [I tried to lose weight. I just don't have the willpower].

Superior people just solve problems. [Some people have succeeded in losing weight. I will study how they did it]." - Epictetus.

<u>Build cognitive reserve</u> by being enthusiastic to learn something everyday, reading at every opportunity, and try to have at least one smart person you can talk to.

If no one wants to talk to you, then write books.

<u>Optimize your environment</u>:

Have a nice, quiet place to study.

Have a nice, quiet place to sleep.

<u>Optimize your kitchen</u>:

Store food in GLASS containers.

Eat off glass plates. If you have to eat off a painted plate, then check it for lead.

Use stainless steel or titanium cookware. Not iron or aluminum.

Do not let aluminum foil touch your food. Do not eat food out of aluminum containers.

Chapter 4

Vitamin C, fruit, and Linus Pauling

Linus Pauling (LP), winner of 2 nobel prizes, took 10-18 grams of vitamin C every day.

One of my biochemistry mentors, Barbara Conrad, was friends with LP. She said, "He's so smart, that talking to him is like talking to three people at the same time."

I read LP's book, "How to live longer, and feel better." LP is fun to read, but he bounces all over the place.

He starts out saying interesting things like, "All amino acids in the human body are in the "L-form" of chiral shape ("L" is "L"evo for "L"eft).

This shape causes cilia to spin like corkscrews in a specific direction… and that's why our liver is on the right side."

Then he says stupid stuff like, "It's proven that high cholesterol is associated with coronary atherosclerosis…. You can eat whatever you want."

That's an obvious contradiction!

The good thing about LP is that he reminded people that vitamin C has lots of benefits, and lots of research behind it; research like that of doctors Cameron, Cathcart, and Klenner.

The bad thing about LP is that he sounds like a vitamin salesman.

Instead of promoting isolated, supplements of sodium ascorbate, he should have been encouraging people to eat more fruits.

I recommend to eat lots of fruits and vegetables — a minimum of 7 servings per day — preferably 10 or more servings per day.

I typically eat 8 on work days, and 30 on nonwork days.

"Mastering diabetes" authors like Cyrus Wombatta and Bobby Bigpoo eat tons of fruits, like 30 or more servings per day.

Almost all animals can make vitamin C, except for primates, humans, fruit bats, and guinea pigs.

It is thought that these "animals" don't make vitamin C, because they don't need to make vitamin C. They get it from their diets.

We are made to eat fruits and plants; this book could have been called, "On the origin of health by selection of plant foods."[16]

Vitamin C is needed for collagen synthesis. Collagen synthesis is needed for wound healing. Better collagen synthesis means better wound healing.

LP says that people with wound healing issues should take high dose vitamin C. I don't know about that.

I would recommend that they eat lots of fruits and vegetables, and avoid things that decrease blood flow.

How to improve blood flow:

Things to do:

- **100% vegan diet** because:

    - **Potassium** is a vasodilator. Plants have potassium.

    - Arugula **salad** and other cruciferous vegetables help to increase Nitric Oxide (vasodilator).

    - Eat **starches** and **fruits** to satisfy hunger.

    - Eat **vegetables** for nutrients.

- **Walk** more. Walking increases nitric oxide. Walking improves venous blood flow. Walking also improves lymph flow.

---

16 Parody of "On the origin of species by natural selection" by Charles Darwin.

- Keep **warm**. Warmth lowers blood viscosity.

- **Sunshine** activates subcutaneous nitric oxide precursors.

- **Sleep** 7-8 hours per night.

- Try to increase **parasympathetic** mood for "rest and digest."

Things to avoid:

- **Sodium** because inhibits nitric oxide.

- **Fructose** because increases uric acid which inhibits nitric oxide —
  more hypertension — more gout.

  - Fructose is only metabolized by the liver, like a toxin.
  - Fructose increase in diet parallels obesity increase.
  - Fructose excess predisposes to elevated cholesterol and fatty
    liver.

- **Fatty liver** because increases uric acid.

- **MSG** because causes addiction to junk food which can lead to
  obesity.
  - Glutamate is an amino acid, and therefore can be called
    "natural flavors."
  - Glutamate is an excitatory neurotransmitter — accounts
    for 70% of brain neurotransmitters.
  - The circumventricular organs — around the third
    ventricle — lack a blood brain barrier.
  - All human amino acids are in the "L" form.
  - Some synthetic MSG has glutamate in the "D" form.
  - The "D" form might be able to bypass splanchnic
    regulation, and thus pass to the brain, where it can be
    neurotoxic.
  - Normally, L-glutamate in sequestered in the gut lining
    cells, so that toxic blood levels are avoided.

- **Tobacco** because causes hypertension and atherosclerosis.

- **Alcohol** because causes fatty liver.
    - Alcohol also causes stiffening of RBC plasma membrane by increasing the percent of saturated fat.
    - Stiff RBC's means elevated blood viscosity.
    - Increased viscosity causes hypertension.
    - Takes more pressure for heart to pump a milkshake (high viscosity blood) than water (normal blood).

- **Excess EDC's** (Endocrine Disrupting Chemicals) like parabens, aluminum, BPA, whole milk.
    - EDC's are in deodorants, moisturizers, sunscreen, laundry detergent, shampoo, perfume.
    - EDC's make a person fat because they trick the hypothalamus, and PPAR gamma receptor into thinking it's pregnant;
    - so the body stores more fat — energy for the baby.

- **Nonorganic foods**, because some herbicides —present in plant and animal foods are estrogenic — and some can cause leaky gut. If you can't afford organic, then it's even more important to be 100% vegan, because feed lot cattle are often fed with herbicide sprayed corn.

- "If there is no organic, then everything is permitted." - Fyodor Dostoevsky.[17]

- **Excess cholesterol** = avoid meat because all animal foods contain cholesterol in every cell membrane. That's how animals rigidify plasma cell membranes.

- **Saturated fat** = avoid meat because animal food is primarily muscle; muscle means protein and saturated fat.

- A useful way to think of meat is as 50:50 food — that's a reasonable approximation. 50% animal protein, and 50% saturated fat. Yikes! Both are bad for you.

- Yes, fish has saturated fat.

---

17 Parody from "Brothers Karamazov" by Dostoevsky, where Ivan had said, "If there is no God, then everything is permitted."

Teach a man to avoid fish,

and you keep him

healthy for life!

- **Avoid trans fats**. Trans fats were first introduced in 1911. The first myocardial infarction in America was reported in 1911.

- The incidence of coronary disease in America has gone up, up, and away, since then — with the graph line ascending at a 45 degree angle — other than brief improvements during rationing in 1918, and the early 1940's.

- The trend toward low fat diets around 1970, also briefly reduced coronary artery disease. Fat diabetics used to be rare. Nowadays, fat diabetics are ubiquitous.

- Trans fats stiffen RBC plasma cell membranes, which decreases RBC deformability. Decreased RBC deformability means increased blood viscosity.

- Gregory Sloop MD — the genius who figured out the major mechanisms of atherosclerosis — has shown that elevated blood viscosity is the unifying feature of almost all atherosclerosis risk factors.

- **Avoid all oils**. Vegetable oils have a lot of omega 6 fats which are inflammatory and atherogenic.

- "What about coconut oil?" Too much saturated fat.

- Oils are liquid fat. Oils are as caloric dense as it gets. A moment on your lips, forever on your hips.

- For most fatsos, quitting oils is one of the fastest ways to lose weight.

- I have a skinny, middle age, doctor friend, who "disappeared" for two months. I asked him, "Where've you been?"

- He said, "I had a myocardial infarction, and almost died."

- I said, "I thought you were vegetarian?"

- He said, "I am. I have no risk factors except for **vegetable oils**."

- ## What about olive oil?

- Yeah, yeah, yeah. The gift of the Greeks. Athena met with Odysseus in Ithaca, under an olive tree; and Odysseus and Penelope built their bed around an olive tree so that it was immovable like their marriage and love.[18]

- It's a beautiful story, but olive oil is still liquid fat. Olive oil in addition to containing monounsaturated fat, also contains around 10% saturated fat.

- Remember what Laocoon said at the gates of Troy, "I fear Greeks, even when bringing gifts."[19]

- Do not let olive oil get past the "gates" of your teeth, that guard your mouth, and your health.

---

18 From "The Oddysey" by Homer.
19 From "The Aeneid" by Virgil..

- "No oil. Not one drop."   - Caldwell Esselstyn MD.

- "What about articles that say saturated fat is okay?"

- Other than arterial occlusion, and mitochondrial dysfunction — the two most common causes of cell death — saturated fat is good for you.

- Try to minimize **psychological stress** because:

    - **Catecholamines** are prothrombotic, and immune supressing (siderophores for bacteria).

    - **Cortisol** is obesogenic, atherogenic, and immuno suppressogenic.

Strong connective tissue-extracellular matrix, made with adequate vitamin C, helps prevent cancer spread according to LP.

LP says that normal ocular, aqueous humor has lots of vitamin C. Low vitamin C in aqueous humor is associated with increased risk of cataracts.

I look at brain CT scans every day, and it's obvious that the same patients who lose their teeth, tend to lose their eyes to cataracts.

Bilateral cataract surgery is a traveling companion of toothless mouths.

Robert Cathcart was an orthopedic surgeon who switched to treating infections, because he was so impressed by vitamin C. Cathcart would titrate vitamin C dosage to just below what causes loose stools. He said this is how the body optimizes it level of vitamin C.

Cathcart, Klenner, Pauling, and other researchers say that the body needs more vitamin C when it is actively healing a wound or fighting an infection.

This variable demand for vitamin C is the reason they recommend much higher doses of vitamin C when a person is acutely ill.

I was amazed at how much literature there is on vitamin C. Doctors like Klenner and Cathcart had patients taking huge doses of vitamin C, like 40-50x higher than expected.

I would be afraid of kidney stones if vitamin C was given on a chronic basis; because sometimes, some vitamin C is metabolized to oxalate.

I do not take any vitamin C supplements. If I had an acute illness, I would just eat more fruit, and salads.

The initial curve relating plasma levels of vitamin C with dietary intake of vitamin C is very steep, until you get to around 400 mg/d. Thus it seems wise to at least eat that much.

Nowadays, humans eat a lot of COOKED starch.

What did humans eat before Prometheus gave them fire?

Probably a lot of FRUIT, and greens, and starchy tubers.

Agriculture became widespread 10,000 years ago.

What did humans eat before agriculture?

Probably a lot of FRUIT! And some starchy tubers, or whatever else was available.

What did our theoretical "primate" ancestors eat?

49

A lot of greens and fruit.

Take a look at a chimp's mouth. They got some big canines. We are more of a plant eater than them.

By the way, I don't think I evolved from a chimp. You might've, but not me.

Supposedly, humans evolved in tropical climates.

Isn't that where there's a lot of FRUIT?

What happens when humans migrate to northern climates?

They eat more meat, and drink more milk.

The eat less fruits and vegetables.

They get more chronic diseases, and more autoimmune diseases.

Why do people in tropical climates get sick?

More infections.

What is the best way to live, for health?

Warm enough. Good plumbing and sanitation. Good food. Good exercise. Good antibiotics. Good social support.

What are good sources of vitamin C?

Fruits in general are good. Kiwi fruit in particular. Apples, berries, cantaloupe, papaya, and oranges are good.

Cabbage, cauliflower, brussel sprouts, and kale have a lot of vitamin C.

Other good foods include potatos,

What foods are poor in vitamin C?

Grains. That's another advantage of fruits.

What are the problems with fruits?

Fruits are more expensive than grains.

Some fruits, like bananas, are too sweet for some people.

Super sweet fruits, like bananas, can cause rebound hypoglycemia.

What else is good about fruit?

Persons with the highest intakes of fruits have higher blood levels of vitamin C , and they have lower risk of coronary artery disease or cancer.

Does fruit have any other advantages?

Yes.

Fruit is lower in protein, than starch. Most people eat way to much protein. Excess protein is bad for the kidneys.

What about acid load?

Grains tend to be slightly acidic. Acid creates extra work for the kidneys.

Fruits tend to be alkaline, which means better for kidneys.

Fruits are a perfect food for protecting the kidneys; high in energy, alkaline, and low in protein.

Your kidneys love fruits!

What do kidneys do?

Kidneys excrete nitrogen in the form of urea.

Protein is the only macronutrient that has nitrogen. Fat and carbohydrate do not have any nitrogen.

Animal foods are protein, fat, and acid.

Plant foods are carbohydrate, fiber and alkali.

Kidneys maintain the blood pH between 7.35 and 7.45.

Why is kidney excretion of nitrogen, and balance of pH a big deal?

Because the kidneys are made for an easy life in a plant based human.

When a human eats a lot of meat — a lot of nitrogen and acid — the kidney has to go into HYPERFILTRATION mode.

What is hyperfiltration?

Hyperfiltration means a lot of increased work for your kidneys. It's like working double shifts, seven days a week.

Chronic hyperfiltration leads to premature kidney failure and death.

What is the RDA for vitamin C?

In adult women its 75 mg/day.

In adult men, it's 90 mg/day.

What do I think of the RDA for vitamin C?

It's kind of a joke. If you eat a lot of fruits, you will get much more vitamin C than that.

If you eat a lot of fruits, you will be much healthier.

Do I take vitamin C supplements?

No.

Would I take a vitamin supplement like sodium ascorbate?

Only if I was really sick, or someone in my family, and not getting better; in that context, I would be willing to try it.

If I were to take vitamin C, which type would I take?

I am not an expert on vitamin C, but so far from my reading, the best type to take is sodium ascorbate.

There might be potassium ascorbate. If other things are equal, I would rather take potassium, than sodium, because potassium is a vasodilator, and sodium is a vasoconstrictor.

Sodium decreases endothelial nitric oxide. Potassium increases endothelial nitric oxide.

I would not take calcium ascorbate, because I worry about that leading to too much calcium ingestion.

I would read about how Cathcart, Klenner, Pauling, and Cameron administered it.

"Ascorbic acid is the safest, and most valuable substance available to the physician."   - Frederic Klenner.

What about vitamin C in pills? In powder? In liposomes? Given IV?

Don't know. Don't know. Don't know.

What other potential benefits with vitamin C?

It might be useful for heavy metal, and halogen detoxification, like with aluminum and mercury, etc.

What about all those studies saying that vitamin C is of no benefit?

Proponents of vitamin C would say that the doses given were too low.

Blah, blah, blah. All this gossipy chatter about vitamin C.

Where's the science?

Most pathogens are oxidants which means that they STEAL ELECTRONS. Pathogens tend to take electrons, and never give them back.

Carbon monoxide steals electrons away from oxygen.

Antioxidants are electron donors. Electron donors are also called "reducing agents." When an atom gains an electron, its valence number goes DOWN, and it is therefore said to be "REDUCED."

Antioxidants give away electrons to quench oxidant pathogens. Vitamin C is a wonderful electron donor.

Antioxidant also means "scavenger of free radicals."

Vitamin C is the most important water soluble, antioxidant in the human body.

Vitamin C is called "A-Scorbic acid." A means without. Scorbic means scurvy. A-scorbic = without scurvy.

English sailors got scurvy, until they ate limes, and then they were called

"Limeys."

Meat is deficient in antioxidants.

Plants are loaded with antioxidants. To be healthy is to be reduced.

To obtain antioxidants, you need to eat plants.

There is a network of antioxidants in the human body that protect it from oxidants. The network of antioxidants includes vitamin C, vitamin E, and glutathione.

Higher plasma concentrations of vitamin C are associated with longer lifespans.

What does vitamin C do for collagen?

Vitamin C is needed for hydroxylation of proline to make hydroxyProline, and of lysine to make hydroxyLysine.

Collagen is a triple helix protein with lots of hydroxyProline and hydroxyLysine.

What about norepinephrine?

Vitamin C is need for conversion of dopamine into norepinephrine by the enzyme dopamine hydroxylase.

What about vitamin C and HIF?

HIF stands for Hypoxia Inducible Factor. HIF increases VEGF (Vascular Endothelial Growth Factor), and initiates angiogenesis, neovascularization.

HIF is activated by hypoxia.

Typically, normoxia (normal oxygen) leads to HIF being **inactivated by vitamin C dependent** hydroxylation enzymes.

When vitamin C is deficient, then HIF is less likely to get turned off.

So what if HIF does not get turned off?

If HIF does not get turned off, then it might persist even under normoxic conditions.

That means, ongoing angiogensis, neovascularization!!!

Cancer cells use neovascularization to increase their ability to metastasize!!!

Vitamin C is also needed to make the extracellular matrix stronger, with better collagen, and this may help to decrease cancer's ability to spread.

Fruit has as much fiber as grains.

One serving of wild, blue berries has 6 grams of fiber; more than oatmeal at 4 grams fiber.

Fruit has lots of vitamin C. The reason humans have color vision is probably so we could recognize when fruits were ripe.

Are you saying that vitamin C deficiency might make it easier for cancer to spread?

Yes. It appears that cancer can spread more readily through "weak" collagen, extracellular matrix;

and that excess neovascularization due to vitamin deficiency might make it easier for cancer to metastasize!!

What about vitamin C and histones?

Epigenetics can regulate DNA transcription by controlling histone methylation.

DNA has a negative charge because of its phosphate backbone.

Histones have a positive charge, which attracts them to DNA.

Methylation of histones neutralizes their positive charge, and thus makes them less attracted to DNA.

When DNA moves away from its histone, the DNA becomes more accessible for RNA transcription, and thus protein synthesis.

Several **HISTONE DEMETHYLASE ENZYMES REQUIRE VITAMIN C**.

When vitamin C is deficient, the affected histones are kept separate from their usual, normally tighter relationship with DNA.

This permits increased DNA transcription, and thus increased protein synthesis.

Cancer needs increased DNA transcription, and protein synthesis, for it to grow, and spread.

Histone hypermethylation is associated with cancer growth.

What about vitamin C, and the DNA itself?

DNA itself (not the histones) can undergo hydroxymethylation.

Hydroxymethylation of DNA itself is also vitamin C dependent via TET (Ten Eleven Translocation enzyme).

Vitamin C deficiency related inability to to hydroxymethylate DNA is associated with increased risk of cancer.

What are the SIX ways that vitamin C might decrease the risk of cancer growth?

1. Stronger **extracellular matrix** collagen might delay cancer spread.

2. **Deactivation of HIF** might delay cancer angiogenesis.

3. **Histone demethylation** might delay unwanted protein synthesis.

4. **DNA hydroxymethylation** might decrease risk of cancer growth.

5. **Scavenging of ROS** to prevent DNA damage, and lipid peroxidation.

6. **Maintenance of nitric oxide levels** which helps prevent tissue atherosclerosis, and hypoxia, and thus helps maintain mitochondrial function.

What about the benefits of fruits for sleep deprivation?

Lack of sleep is perceived as psychological stress.

When sleep deprived, we crave sweets.

This craving is usually satisfied by drinking coffee, and eating cookies or donuts; which is a nutritional mistake.

Our body really craves FRUITS!!

Junk food like cookies and donuts did not even exist when human biochemical pathways were developed.

What about the immune system?

Macrophages and lymphocytes concentrate vitamin C up to 100 fold, more than the amount in plasma.

Adequate levels of vitamin C improve immune system function.

Vitamin C helps to limit inflammation to the minimal amount necessary for healing, and to avoid damage to adjacent tissues;

in other words, vitamin C helps to "clean up" after inflammation, so that your normal tissues are not injured by the inflammation.

What about vitamin C and nitric oxide?

Vitamin C helps maintain TetraHydroBiopterin which is needed for synthesis of nitric oxide in endothelial cells.

Nitric oxide is the most important vasodilator for arteries.

Lack of nitric oxide is associated with vasoconstriction, hypertension, and atherosclerosis.

Therefore, vitamin C helps to prevent atherosclerosis.

What about vitamin C and prevention of lipid peroxidation?

Vitamin C is part of a network of antioxidants that includes vitamin E and glutathione.

Vitamin E is lipid soluble, and located inside membranes. Vitamin E quenches lipid peroxidation chain reactions in membranes.

Vitamin C is water soluble, and therefore typically located in the aqueous environment of the cell cytoplasm;

but vitamin C can go to the edge of membranes the lipid water interface — and help regenerate the reduced form of vitamin E (so that vitamin E can get back to work quenching free radical, lipid peroxidation).

What is the chemical structure of vitamin C?

In most animals, vitamin C is synthesized from glucose; and vitamin C's structure is similar to glucose. Vitamin C is a 5 member ring with 4 carbons and 1 oxygen with 1 ketone, and 2 hydroxy groups, and one carbon-carbon double bond.

Where can you learn more about vitamin C?

Textbooks of nutritional biochemistry have summaries of vitamin C related reactions.

Study Pauling, Cathcart, and Klenner to get started. Then you will learn about the other experts on vitamin C.

Take home message:

Eat MORE fruits to get vitamin C!

Eat more fruits to improve your energy level.

Eat more fruits to lower your risk of obesity, diabetes, hypertension, and cancer.

Fruits are the perfect food to protect kidney function: high energy, alkaline, and low protein.

References:

Pauling, Linus. Book. "How to live longer, and feel better." (Paperback book).

Klenner, Frederic (1971) Observations on the dose, and administration of ascorbic acid. Journal of applied nutrition. 23 (3&4): 61-88.

Klenner, Frederic (April 1951) Massive doses of vitamin C and diseases. Southern medicine and surgery. 103(4): 101-107.

Cathcart, Robert (1981) Vitamin C. Titrating to bowel tolerance. Medical hypotheses 7(11):1359-1376.

Chapter 5

Telomeres, Aging, and Hayflick

Do you know what the Hayflick limit is?

Dr Hayflick was a researcher, in the mid 1900's, working with human fetal tissue cultures.

Hayflick noticed that human, somatic cells —somatic means "body," as in the body line of cells — and not the germ line of cells as in eggs or sperm = germ cells) — typically could only divide about 60 times, and then they died.

Hayflick put human tissue culture cells into a refrigerator for extended amounts of time.

When the cells were taken out of the fridge, and rewarmed, they REMEMBERED their intrinsic Hayflick limit.

Hayflick's observation became known as the Hayflick limit.

Dr Hayflick did not know why the cells had a Hayflick limit, or how they were able to remember it, even after a prolonged time in the fridge.

By 1960, the Hayflick limit was published and known by the scientific community. Dr Hayflick had shown that typical, normal, somatic cells are not immortal.

Why is Hayflick limit a big deal?

With science, the truth is approached asymptotically. The concept of the Hayflick limit gives us a useful way to delay aging.

Anything that delays reaching the Hayflick limit makes us live longer.

Anything that speeds up reaching the Hayflick limit makes us die sooner.

What causes the Hayflick limit?

The answer comes from DNA structure and replication. DNA is a long polymer of nucleotides called a chromosome.

The end of a chromosome is called a telomere. Telomeres are like the end of a shoelace where there's a tight plastic wrap.

Telomeres have a bunch of repeating sequences of DNA — like TTAGG — that signal the physical endpoint of the chromosome.

When a cell replicates, the DNA has to be copied. The DNA double helix opens up like a two "rail" train track being pulled into a letter "Y" shape.

The first "rail" is called the leading strand, and it proceeds in a straight line, inwards, along the replication fork. The leading strand is easily copied in continuous fashion by the DNA polymerase enzyme.

The second "rail" is called the lagging strand. The lagging strand is replicated in the **OPPOSITE** direction of the leading strand.

The lagging strand is replicated in staggered steps, because DNA polymerase cannot attach to the original template DNA strand, until an RNA primer has been laid down first.

The lagging strand runs into a problem at the telomere, because the RNA polymerase can't attach to the end of the telomere.

So the **end of the telomere on the lagging strand cannot be copied!**

Inability to copy the end of the telomere on the lagging strand means that with every cell replication, the **CHROMOSOME GETS SHORTER!**

Eventually, this cell replication related chromosome shortening progresses to the extent that important DNA gene(s) — that the cell needs to survive — are lost.

Now the cell becomes dysfunctional, and then dies relatively soon.

How does knowledge of telomeres help us to delay aging?

Some foods stimulate cell proliferation. Animal protein increases **ILGF** (Insulin Like Growth Factor), and this may accelerate the rate at which the Hayflick limit is reached.

Saturated fat causes insulin resistance, which leads to increased insulin levels in the blood. Insulin is an anabolic hormone.

Elevated **insulin** may accelerate the rate at which some cells reach the Hayflick limit. Insulin itself is a growth factor.

Meat contains relatively large amounts of the branched chain amino acid, leucine. **Leucine stimulates mTOR**. MTOR is one of the master regulatory systems for cell growth.

When mTOR senses that amino acids-nutrients, like leucine, are abundant, it tells cells, that now is a good time to grow and proliferate.

Meat increases estrogen reabsorption in the gut, and this increases blood estrogen levels. Higher blood levels of estrogen stimulates growth of cells in the breast, uterus, and prostate.

When a young man takes a piss, he just takes a piss; it only takes a minute.

65

A middle age man has to ask his prostate for permission first; it takes about 5 minutes.

I always have a book in the bathroom, so I can read while I'm waiting for prostate permission. I read a book a week in that way.

What's the point?

A young weightlifter might like to eat food that stimulates growth, so his muscles can get bigger faster.

After 40, you don't want growth stimulators because they might accelerate aging by rushing you to the Hayflick limit.

Worse yet, these growth stimulators might tip the balance in cancer cells towards proliferation.

Everybody has some dormant cancer cells in their body. It typically takes decades for a clone of cancer cells to become clinically relevant.

The smart move is to AVOID MEAT so you lower your risk of premature aging, premature cancer, and premature death.

Is there anything else worth knowing about the Hayflick limit and telomeres?

Yes. Dr Elizabeth Blackburn won a nobel prize for discovering the enzyme called "telomerase."

Telomerase enzyme rebuilds telomeres. Rebuilding telomeres enables a cell to become IMMORTAL.

Stem cells have telomerase. Cancer cells have telomerase.

Dr Hayflick says that the most unique thing about cancer cells is that they make telomerase enzyme.

So what? How is that helpful?

Dr Blackburn teamed up with Dr Dean Ornish to study what lengthens telomeres (slows aging), and what shortens telomeres (accelerates aging).

Blackburn and Ornish found that telomeres were shortened by cigarette smoking.

They also found that excess, psychological stress caused telomere shortening.

Low fat, whole food, vegan diet causes **telomere lengthening!**

Take home points:

Avoid meat so you can avoid growth stimulators that might accelerate the rate at which you reach the Hayflick limit.

Minimize psychological stress to the extent you can.

Chapter 6

Jose can you SEE with this diet

I've seen many thousands of brain MRI's and CT's.

Whenever a patient's brain is full of atherosclerosis;

they usually also have **C**ataracts or **D**iabetic retinopathy or "**A**ge" related macular degeneration or **H**ypertensive retinopathy or **G**laucoma, or all of the above (**C-DAHG**).

What a way to go through the golden years, cognitive impaired, and vision impaired.

Diseases that travel together usually have a similar cause.

Notice that **C-DAHG are all dietary diseases!**

To my eyes, C-DAHG diseases are just variations on a theme: like a fractal;

like Johann Sebastian Bach's "Art of the Fugue" in the key of LDL major.

C-DAHG are the most common causes of blindness in middle age and older adults.

Years ago, I noticed that patients with cerebral amyloid angiopathy (CAA) which is a disease characterized by brain hemorrhages; also often had hemorrhagic, hypertensive retinopathy, or diabetic retinopathy.

I had a vision that these diseases were related.

Several papers have now confirmed that association. I also noticed that the pattern of brain hemorrhages from CAA, often overlapped with those from hypertension.

In fact, neuroradiologists often cannot distinguish old brain bleeds from CAA, from those due to hypertension.

Whenever two diseases look the SAME, one has to consider that they are the SAME.

Do you see where this is going?

The SAME patients often are obese, and hypertensive, and diabetic.

Obesity is associated with hypertension and diabetes. Hypertension and diabetes are associated with hemorrhagic retinopathy.

What about atherosclerosis?

Hypertension and diabetes cause atherosclerosis. Atherosclerosis causes dry AMD (Age related Macular Degeneration), and wet AMD.

What causes macular degeneration?

The fovea is the part of the eye with lots of cone type photoreceptors, and high visual acuity. The macula is the center of the fovea, and the site of highest visual acuity.

Nature in her wisdom, did not put blood vessels inside the fovea, because blood vessels would lower visual acuity.

When a person has normal arteries and capillaries, it's easy for the fovea to get enough blood supply, by diffusion from the nearby capillaries, in the choroid.

Our ancestors didn't have atherosclerosis, because they didn't drink fructose, or eat processed food, and they ate very little meat.

Now we all know that saturated fat causes elevated LDL cholesterol, leading to RBC rouleaux, and atherosclerosis.

Saturated fat also causes mitochondrial dysfunction via reversal of electron transport, which leads to insulin resistance and diabetes. Hyperglycemia then leads to diabetic retinopathy.

Hyperglycemia decreases WBC chemotaxis and activation which causes **immunosuppression**.

It is less widely known that PUFA's (PolyUnsaturated Fatty Acids also cause mitochondrial dysfunction.

What is the nomenclature for fatty acids?

Fatty acids have two ends. The carboxylic acid carbon is also called a carbonyl carbon. The methyl terminal carbon is called the omega carbon.

Omega 6 means that the first double bond begins on carbon number six, counting from the omega end of the fatty acid.

The typical omega 6 fatty acid has its first double bond on carbon number 6, and then its second on carbon number 9. The C8 carbon in between the double bonds is a methylene group CH2.

The C8 methylene carbon between the omega 6 & 9 double bonds is called a "methylene bridge."

The methylene bridge carbon has a relatively weak bond to its hydrogen.

70

This weak carbon–hydrogen bond makes it vulnerable to reacting with free radicals like superoxide.

Omega 6 PUFA's are highly vulnerable to free radical induced lipid peroxidation. Lipid peroxidation is rare in saturated fat.

Lipid peroxidation can initiate a chain reaction that destroys multiple fatty acids in a cell membrane.

Lipid peroxidation of mitochondrial membranes can lead to uncoupling of electron transport, and oxidative phosphorylation — similar to what happens with brown fat — and an inability of the mitochondria to generate energy.

Lipid peroxidation of plasma cell membranes can lead to cell death.

This same risk of lipid peroxidation is associated the fact that omega 3 and omega 6 oils can become rancid.

Free, unliganded iron in the cytoplasm can lead to autocatalytic Fenton and Haber Weiss reactions with the generation of many reactive oxygen species (ROS) — free radicals.

These ROS cause increased risk of lipid peroxidation, and ferroptosis.

What about omega 6 PUFA's?

Dietary **omega 6** PUFA's like **linoleic** acid (LA), (C18:2, n6,9) tend to get elongated into arachidonic acid. Metabolism of arachidonic acid — called the "omega 6 pathway" — tends to produce proinflammatory chemicals. Junk food, and meat are sources of arachidonic acid. Most meats are abundant sources of arachidonic acid, especially chicken and eggs. Plant foods have relatively little arachidonic acid.

The same enzymes used to elongate omega 6 fatty acids are used to elongate omega 3 fatty acids, and there is a limited amount of these enzymes. If omega 6 fatty acids are present in excessive amounts, then they tend to crowd out the omega 3 fatty acids.

Meaty, sweety, oily humans are often relatively deficient in **omega 3** fatty acids. Plants contain omega 3 fatty acids like alpha-**linoleic** acid (ALA), which can be made into EPA and DHA.

Omega 3 PUFA's go through the "omega 3 pathway," which is relatively anti-inflammatory.

Inexperienced people think that saturated fat is much worse than omega 6 PUFA's. In reality, they're both bad.

People used to think that omega 6 PUFA's weren't that bad, because they don't increase LDL cholesterol, as much as saturated fat does.

David Blankenthorn's research, and Nathan Pritikin's, and Caldwell Esselstyn's study of the nutrition literature showed that PUFA's are also major contributers to causing atherosclerosis.

What about atherosclerosis in AMD?

Atherosclerosis, and RBC rouleaux cause hypoxia of the macula. Hypoxia leads to increased HIF (Hypoxia Inducible Factor).

HIF leads to increased VEGF (Vascular Endothelial Growth Factor). VEGF leads to neovascularization.

Neovascularization covers up, and damages the macula photoreceptor cones, which causes decreased visual acuity.

The neovascular vessels are fragile, and can leak fluid, or bleed, leading to sudden loss of visual acuity.

What about glaucoma?

High blood pressure is associated with high intraocular pressure and development of glaucoma. Glaucoma is the most common cause of blindness in African Americans.

Increased intraocular pressure can compress the optic nerve, and cause blindness. Glaucoma might begin with peripheral vision loss, that is initially ignored.

What about cataracts?

Diets and lifestyles that cause atherosclerosis also cause cataracts. High fat, meat sweet diets tend to be low in vitamin C. Low levels of vitamin C increase the risk for cataracts.

Cataracts are associated with low vitamin C. Vitamin C deficiency is associated with weak collagen. Weak collagen is associated with teeth falling out.

Thousands of times, I've seen that the same patient who has bilateral cataract surgery, has also lost all his teeth.

Milk sugar, lactose, specifically the galactose component, is also associated with increased risk of cataracts.

Just because someone retains the enzyme to split lactose into glucose and galactose, does not automatically mean they have the enzymes to metabolize galactose.

In the 1930's, a dentist, named Weston Price, traveled around the world to correlate diet with dentition. Dr Price observed that populations eating their old fashioned, endemic, plant based diets had good teeth.

The populations that had switched to eating modern junk food with refined flour, oils, and added sugar, had poor dentition.

What does this have to do with the brain?

The eye is innervated by cranial nerve number two, and the retina is considered part of the brain.

The eye is more than the window to the soul; the eye is the window to the brain.

What about the anatomy of the eye and the brain?

Retinal rods and cones are like neurons in the brain. Rods and cones — like cortical neurons — have super high metabolic rates; they eat lots of glucose; you can see them light up on a PET (Positive Emmision Tomography) scan, due to high glucose uptake.

Retinal pigmented epithelium "support cells," are like glial "support cells" in the brain. The retinal pigmented epithelium of the eye, functions like the glymphatic system of the brain; it cleans up at night.

Bruch's membrane in the eye — between the choroid and the fovea — is like the blood brain barrier in the brain.

What is the overlapping mechanism of disease in the eye and the brain?

Dry macular degeneration is due to ischemic atrophy of the fovea.

74

If a patient has ischemic damage of the eye, you can bet they've got ischemic damage of the brain.

If they've got hypertensive damage of the eye, they've got hypertensive damage of the brain.

If they've got antioxidant deficiency — vitamin C deficiency — cataracts — in the eye, they've got oxidative stress and neuro degeneration in the brain.

Researchers in the 1960's got an 80x magnification microscope to look at the eyeball. Then they fed the patients a high fat meal, and they could see the small arteries in the back of the eye OCCLUDING!!

Most of these arteries reopened, but not all of them. You can bet your bippy that the same thing happens in the brain. This has been shown in mouse studies.

In a future chapter we'll talk more about why brains shrink (atrophy), and how brain shrinkage can be minimized (no pun intended).

Take home message:

Master bay shun is not the most common cause of blindness. Diet related atherosclerosis variations are the most common causes of blindness.

C-DAHG are all dietary diseases that occur in eaters of meat, oils, and processed foods.

In the Bible, one reads about healing the blind so they can see; and it's a miracle, and one wonders is this allegorical.

What if it were possible to reverse blindness in the

75

real world?

Complete blindness is unlikely to be reversible.

Partial blindness is sometimes partially reversible.

Back in the 1940's Dr Kempner showed reversal of proliferative retinopathies by putting patients on a 100% plant, low salt, low fat, predominantly rice based diet.

What's good for you heart is good for your brain, and your eyes.

Eat a low salt, low fat, whole food, vegan diet and you:

- Prevent atherosclerosis, so you reduce risk of AMD.

- Have plenty of vitamin C, so you reduce risk of cataracts.

- Prevent HTN, so you reduce risk of glaucoma.

- Have lots of antioxidants, and very little omega 6 fats, so you reduce risk of lipid peroxidation.

Chapter 7

Milk is a Mis-aster

Milk is a Mistake + disaster = Mis-aster.

The halo around the milk carton is gone.

To be fair, milk has never caused me any problems that I'm aware of.

In college, at Stanford, I lived in the best athlete fraternity, and we all drank milk, and considered it a helpful part of our nutrition.

We never tested that assumption by reading, or comparing it to other diets.

I drank 12-16 ounces of skim milk everyday with cereal until 45 years old, and then every other day between 45-55, and none after that.

I became a lacto-vegetarian at 40 years old, and a 100% vegan at 55 years old.

The side effects of lactose are unique to milk; the remaining problems are about the same with other types of meat.

The reason for an entire chapter on milk is that it was such an emotional shock to learn about the associations of milk with disease.

It's like finding out that the lady you're dating is a prostitute, and even though she seemed so pretty, and so nice, you have to run for your life.

What's bad about milk?

Milk how doth thou disappoint me, let me count the ways.

- Milk is liquid meat.

- Meat has no fiber, so high milk intake can be associated with constipation.

- Saturated fat.

- High estrogen.

- Galactose.

- High calcium. Contrary to popular belief, high dietary calcium is not good for you.

- Milk might be associated with enlargment of tonsils.

- Association with autoimmune disease.

- Association with infertility.

- Animal protein (this is the worst problem).

Why is milk bad for children?

No animal in nature drinks milk after it is weaned.

No animal in nature drinks the milk of another species.

Eating dairy appears to increase the risk of acne.

Infants who drink milk have an increased risk of type one diabetes.

If anyone in your family has type one diabetes, then do NOT give your kid milk.

Ideally, a women should breast feed for 3-4 years — that's what hunter gatherers do.

Obviously, most modern women work, so you gotta feed the kid something else than breast milk.

It's not easy to choose. Cow's milk is associated with type one diabetes.

Added omega 3's are often contaminated with pollutants.

Tap water is routinely not adequately filtered of estrogenics, and other chemicals you don't want for your kid.

If you drink filtered water, you need to check the TDS (Total Dissolved Solids) so you can get an idea of the relative osmolality.

I ALWAYS EAT FIRST, and then only drink water at the end of a meal; so the water will mix with the food. If you drink low osmolality water with an empty stomach, that can have an osmolatity effect on your blood.

Soy is super complicated.

If I was a billionaire, I would get a wet nurse for the kid, and one for myself.

For everyone else, I recommend to read what the great vegan experts like John Mcdougall MD, Neal Barnard MD, and others have to say about it; and don't trust any that are trying to sell you any food or drink.

How could milk have anything to do with type one diabetes?

The mechanism might be "leaky gut."

With leaky gut, relatively large pieces of animal protein can pass from the gut, into the blood.

The animal protein sequences are recognized by our immune systems as foreign.

The animal protein is different enough to be recognized as foreign, but similar enough to mimic human protein sequences.

This similarity is called "molecular mimicry."

Why is molecular mimicry a big deal?

Molecular mimicry is a big deal, because the antibodies to the animal protein can "cross react," and attack the person's own body.

What is antibody "cross reactivity"?

Antibody cross reactivity is when a person's own antibodies react against themselves.

Antibody cross reactivity is one of the major mechanisms of autoimmune disease.

What about milk and premature puberty?

Milk cows are often pregnant. Pregnant cows have high estrogen levels. The estrogen gets into the milk.

Estrogen stimulates proliferation of mammary glands in the breast. Estrogen activates maturation of the uterus.

Girls who drink high estrogen milk are at risk for premature puberty. Premature puberty is amazingly common.

Why is milk bad for men over 40?

Whole milk, 2% and 1% are definite no-no's because TOO MUCH fat and too much estrogen.

Nowadays, the cows are engineered to make milk while they are PREGNANT!

PREGNANT cows have high ESTROGEN.

High estrogen tricks your body into thinking it's pregnant and needs to store weight for the baby.

High estrogen resets the PPAR gamma "fat switch," to store more fat. Drink dairy and you get a big derriere.

Percent of calories from fat:

- Whole cow's milk = 64%

- Low fat, 2% milk = 35%
- 1% milk = 18%
- Cheese = 70%

Even 1% milk has lots of fat.

One cup — (8 ounces) — of whole milk has 8 grams of total fat, and 5 grams of saturated fat.

Increased dietary fat means increased obesity, hypertension, atherosclerosis, and diabetes.

Saturated fat is a major risk factor for type 2 diabetes.

Saturated fat can cause reversal of electron transport in mitochondria. Reversal of electron transport leads to increased production of reactive oxygen species (ROS) like superoxide anions.

Excess superoxide anions can lead to release of some Fe^{2+} (iron) from ferritin.   This unliganded iron can lead to the formation of more ROS.

What about milk's effect on adult women?

Milk might have a harmful effect on ovaries.

Milk might decrease the likelihood that a woman will ovulate, leading to infertility.

Milk consumption is associated with increased risk of autoimmune disease.

What about milk and the risk of cancer in women?

Drinking milk increases the risk of breast cancer.

Milk appears to increase the risk of ovarian cancer.

How does milk increase the risk of ovarian cancer?

Milk sugar is lactose. Lactose is a disaccharide dimer of glucose and galactose.

It appears that galactose is sometimes toxic to ovaries.

Just because a person has the enzyme lactase that enables them to split lactose into glucose and galactose;

that does NOT mean they can metabolize galactose!

What about galactose and the eyes?

Galactose appears to increase the risk of cataracts.

What about breast cancer?

Estrogen stimulates proliferation of breast cells, and uterus cells.

Normal levels of estrogen are part of good health.

Abnormally elevated levels of estrogen cause increased risk of breast cancer and endometrial cancer.

What about fibroids?

Fibroids are benign tumors of the uterus.

Fibroids can cause dysfunctional uterine bleeding. Fibroids are a common reason for hysterectomy.

A lot of people talk about hysterectomies like it's no big deal, a routine rite of passage for a woman. Wrong!!

Women are protected by menstruation, which serves as a therapeutic phlebotomy. That's why women have a 10-15 year advantage on men with before they get SYMPTOMATIC atherosclerosis.

When RBC's (Red Blood Cells) first come out of the bone marrow, they are more flexible = more deformable. Increased RBC flexibility means lowered blood viscosity.

The number of RBC's in blood is called the hematocrit. Hematocrit is the main determinant of how thick the blood is. Blood thickness is called "viscosity."

Monthly menstruation leads a a lower hematocrit, and thus to lower blood viscosity.

Lowered blood viscosity means lowered blood pressure. Lowered blood pressure means less atherosclerosis. Less atherosclerosis means less risk of myocardial infarction, and stroke.

Do hysterectomies increase the risk of dementia?

Sometimes.

Women who get a hysterectomy in their 30's or 40's stop menstruating; these women now have an accelerated risk for atherosclerosis;

and they are at increased risk for **vascular cognitive impairment** (VCI), and dementia.

Whenever I see female 45 - 60 years old with multiple small strokes, the most common reason was hysterectomy in her late 30's or early 40's, and associated hypertension.

Early age hysterectomy also puts a woman at increased risk for congestive heart failure, coronary artery disease, and obesity.

The most common reason for early age hysterectomies include fibroids, and endometriosis.

The Mayo Clinic followed over 2,000 women with hysterectomies, and said that if less than 35 years of age, the woman had a big increase in morbidity, as described above.

I say, that she now needs to be more careful about her atherosclerosis risk factors because her blood is thicker, and she is now at increased risk for iron overload.

There was no change in morbidity if the woman was 50 years of age, or older.

What about migraine headaches?

In some persons, milk can lead to migraine headaches.

MSG is another seldom recognized cause of migraine headaches.

What about autoimmune diseases in adults?

Autoimmune diseases include multiple sclerosis, lupus, rheumatoid arthritis, Hashimoto's thyroiditis, and Sjogren's syndrome.

Type one diabetes can also have an adult onset.

Autoimmune diseases are more common in northern populations.

Why is autoimmune disease more common up north?

The reason for Northern populations to have increased autoimmune disease are thought to be:

Less vitamin D because less sunshine. Sunshine is the best way to maintain vitamin D levels. Dietary vitamin D is not as effective as sunshine obtained vitamin D.

Vitamin D is hydroxylated in the liver to become 25-hydroxy-vitamin D. This liver form of vitamin D is the one usually measured in the blood.

However, the 25-vitamin D then goes to the kidneys for another hydroxylation.

The kidney's hydroxylate vitamin D to 1, 25 – DiHydroxy-vitamin D. The **1,25-vitamin D** is by far the most powerful and important version of vitamin D.

Increased dietary calcium causes inhibition of kidney hydroxylation of 25-vitamin D. Therefore, increased **dietary calcium decreases vitamin D activity**.

Milk has a lot of calcium. Milk calcium decreases production of the 1,25 activated form of vitamin D.

Who cares if dietary calcium decreases vitamin D activity?

In addition to maintaining blood levels of calcium, vitamin D has other important functions.

1,25-vitamin D also helps prevent autoimmune disease!

Are there any other reasons that northern populations have increased autoimmune disease?

Meat is associated with leaky gut. Leaky gut is associated with "molecular mimicry," and antibody "cross reactivity."

Does milk have any effect on cancer in men?

The male prostate is similar to the female uterus.

Increased estrogen is associated with increased risk of benign prostate hypertrophy (BPH), which is the male equivalent of fibroids.

Increased estrogen is associated with increased risk of prostate cancer, which is the male equivalent of endometrial cancer.

What is the scientific evidence that milk is associated with increased risk for prostate cancer?

There are several studies showing increased milk, and increased prostate cancer risk.

The Dean Ornish MD study showed improved outcomes in patients with prostate cancer who went on a vegan diet.

What about the testicles?

Testicular cancer is rare in comparison to prostate cancer.

The scary thing about testicular cancer is that it occurs in relatively younger men, and the treatment routinely includes orchiectomy — removal of a testicle.

Given that milk appears to have a negative effect on ovaries, it is not surprising that milk appears to have a negative effect on testicles.

There is some evidence that eating dairy products like cheese might lower sperm counts.

What about skim milk?

Skim milk avoids the problems associated with fat.

I drank skim milk all my life up to 55 years of age, and I never had a problem from it.

I used to think skim milk was good, because I was lifting weights, and I wanted the protein in milk, but not the fat.

What changed your attitude to milk?

It turns out that animal protein is a problem by itself.

Even skim milk is a problem because of the excess animal protein, and the galactose.

Why is animal protein bad?

Eating animal protein is associated with increased cancer risk in multiple ways.

Animal protein increases **ILGF** (Insulin Like Growth Factor). Increased ILGF is associated with **increased cancer risk**.

Animal protein **increases blood cholesterol**. That is not a misprint. Animal protein increases blood cholesterol, and the risk of atherosclerosis.

Animal protein has increased **methionine**, a sulfur containing amino acid.

During degradation of methionine, the sulfur group can get converted into sulfuric acid, leading to **metabolic acidosis**.

The metabolic acidosis in the blood has to be buffered. The body buffers the blood pH by taking calcium from bones.

Then the calcium is voided by the kidneys. This buffer related calcium causes **CALCIURIA** which means increased urine calcium.

Caffeine causes a small increase in urinary calcium excretion, about 3 mg of calcium loss per serving.

Elevated dietary sodium also causes increased urinary calcium excretion. It has been estimated that each dietary, extra, 1,000 mg intake of sodium, is associated with a loss of 20 mg of calcium into the urine.

Calciuria increases the risk of **kidney stones**. The calcium accumulation in the kidney also worsens kidney function.

Increased blood pressure also causes increased urinary excretion of calcium.

Meat is the main thing to avoid, but **if you are at risk for kidney stones**, it is beneficial to also **avoid caffeine, and sodium**.

Potassium prevents calcium loss in the urine. Potassium dilates arteries. Potassium is high in plant foods, and low in animal foods.

Animal protein burdens the kidneys with excess nitrogen and acid, which puts the kidneys into **HYPERfiltration** mode which accelerates aging of the kidneys.

Are you talking about all animal protein, or just about milk protein?

In general, all animal protein tends to have relatively high methionine levels.

Cow's milk has three times as much protein as human milk. Cow's milk is for cows. Human breast milk is for human babies.

Adult people are better off if they don't drink milk.

The point was that I used to drink milk, because I wanted a source of protein, without fat.

I do not drink milk anymore, at all, because I have learned that animal protein increases my risk for prostate cancer, and other types of cancer.

I also worry about the galactose related risks of cataracts, and for potentially lowering sperm counts.

Besides ILGF and methionine, how else does animal protein increase cancer risk?

Animal protein also tends to be high in leucine. **Leucine** is a major activator of **mTOR**. MTOR is a nutrient sensing system, and a growth regulator.

When nutrients in general — and leucine in particular are available — mTOR tends to signal for increased growth and proliferation.

The concern is that activation of mTOR can stimulate cell growth, and that it might accelerate you towards the **Hayflick limit**, or cancer.

What about people saying that animal protein is "better" than plant protein?

If you are a twenty year old weightlifter, then you might want to eat some meat or drink some skim milk; the animal protein will have more leucine to activate mTOR; and will cause more elevation of ILGF.

The animal protein should be from an animal food, and not from a supplement.

However, if you're over 30 years of age, then the problems outweigh the benefits.

Animal protein is strongly associated with multiple, common, bad diseases like kidney failure, kidney stones, heart disease, stroke, and cancer.

Is it okay for young men who lift weights to take protein supplements?

No! Check out consumer reports from 2012 on protein supplements.

These protein supplements sometimes have poor quality control, and may contain heavy metal contaminants.

These protein supplements often contain animal protein, and impose a heavy workload on the kidneys.

I would NEVER take a protein supplement, because of fear of damaging the kidneys.

Young men love lifting weights; they glory in their high testosterone. Young guys don't know anything, but they are very strong.

To me, a young guy is kind of like a Tyrannosauras Rex dinosaur; you can't learn much from them, but you have to treat them with respect, because they could beat the sh_t out of you.

*"There are no **prudent** young people. Prudence is concerned with specifics as well as universals. Specifics become known from experience, but young*

Lots of young guys take protein supplements, and creatine, and drink all kinds of bizarre energy drinks.

Lots of young guys trash their kidneys.

According to one paper, the average lifespan of a professional bodybuilder is 47 years. That's worse than the average lifespan of a pro football player at 54 years.

Look what happened to Andy Bolton, the first man to deadlift over 1,000 pounds. He ended up in kidney failure, on dialysis, in his mid 40's.

The smart move is to become a 100% low fat, low salt, whole food vegan — to protect the kidneys and all the other body parts — which all benefit from better blood flow; you might be a little bit less strong, but you will maintain good endurance, and sexual potency for much longer, potentially a couple extra decades.

Protein supplements will probably contain large amounts of methionine, and leucine, and be associated with increased cancer risk.

Obviously, I'm jealous of young guys. They're energetic and strong, and they don't have wives. They're relatively free. Even their ignorance has a positive side. They have a naive optimism.

Isn't this chapter a little unfair? Aren't you picking on milk more than other types of meat?

For the last 17 years, I have avoided all forms of meat, except for milk. I used to think milk was the lone angel, out of all the animal foods.

I have always considered milk to be the best option amongst animal foods.

However, now that I have learned more about:

- the increased risk of acne,

- the harmful effects of dietary calcium on vitamin D activation,

- the increased risk of autoimmune disease including hypothyroidism, and type one diabetes,

- that some people don't present with type one diabetes until they are adults,

- the harmful effects of animal protein,

- the increased ILGF,

- and methionine,

- and leucine

- and the increased risk of prostate cancer.

This information led me to decide to never drink milk again.

What about raw milk?

The concern is for risk of bovine tuberculosis.

What about non-organic milk?

Nonorganic milk is also a no-no.

Concern about growth hormone, and contaminants like pesticides and antibiotics.

How to quit dairy

- If drink coffee, drink it black.

- NEVER drink milk as a beverage.

- If eat oatmeal, make it with water.

- Cereals have too much sodium, MSG, and iron. Good to quit eating cereals.

Most people who ditch dairy, go with almond milk.

Neal Barnard MD, one of the best nutrition doctors in the world, uses almond milk.

If you choose almond milk, I recommend to get organic, and to **avoid CYANOcobalamin,** and avoid carageenan.

Unsweetened is better.

I do NOT drink almond milk.

I have no need for it.

I do not drink any type of milk or milk substitute. I do not eat anything associated with dairy.

The only thing I used to use milk for was **cereals**, but ALL the cereals I checked were bad because of sodium, MSG, iron, flax, or other additives.

So I quit eating cereals.

Some people recommend **oat milk**. Oat milk tastes good, but the brand I tried was not refrigerated which makes me wonder about preservatives; and the container had an **aluminum** lining.

I **NEVER** eat food that contacts aluminum because of its association with breast cancer — and therefore likely with prostate cancer — and with Alzheimer's disease.

I tried "skim" **soy milk**, and I got arthritis in my hands — that went away as soon as I quit the soy milk.

Soy is complicated — perhaps the most unusual, and complicated food. Soy can be processed in so many ways. Soy protein is relatively unique. If you want to try soy, make sure you study it a lot, and the old fashioned, least processed versions are likely best. I just avoid soy completely.

Chapter 8

Diabetes

Sung to the tune of "Frere Jaques."

- Frere Jaques, Frere Jaques
  - Dormez vous,
  - dormez vous?

- Sonnez les matines, sonnez les matines!
  - Din, din, don,
  - Din, din, don

- Di-a-be-tes, di-a-be-tes,
- Are you sleeping, are you sleeping?
  - Read a book,
  - read a book!

- Help yourself, help yourself.
  - Don't be a ding dong,
  - Don't be a ding dong,

- Who keeps eating,
- Who keeps eating
  - meat and oils,
  - meat and oils.

What is the most important thing to know about type 2 diabetes?

Diabetes is a LIPID disease.

Diabetes is NOT a carbohydrate disease.

SATurated Fat Causes Insulin Resistance!!!

Insulin resistance leads to hyperglycemia.

Hyperglycemia leads to retinopathy, nephropathy, neuropathy, and microvasculopathy.

To optimize a dietary approach for diabetes, you need to know that fruits and starch are your friend, and that saturated fat is your opponent.

At what age should a person switch to becoming a vegan?

The sooner the better.

The longer a person has type 2 diabetes, the higher their risk of beta cell burnout.

Once the pancreas loses its beta cells, the patient will be permanently insulin dependent.

Who gets diabetes?

Low fat vegans almost never get type 2 diabetes.

People who eat a high fat diet tend to get diabetes. Meat has lots of saturated fat.

Meaties get diabetes. The road to diabetes is paved with meat.
Just one serving of meat per week is associated with a 74% increased risk of type two diabetes.

Plant based populations almost never have diabetes.

When these populations switch to eating the MOFU (Meat, Oils, Fructose, Unknown additives) they start getting type 2 diabetes.

Look what happened in Japan and China. When they ate mostly rice, they were mostly healthy.

Now they are eating more meat and oils, and they have more obesity, and diabetes.

Ditto for the PIMA who were healthy, before they switched to the SAD (Standard American Diet) diet.
The Tarahumara stayed with their old plant based diet, and they are famous for being slim, trim, long distance runners.

Since when has it been known that fat causes insulin resistance?

Since the 1920's. Sweeney's paper in 1927 was called, "Dietary factors that influence the dextrose tolerance test."

Nowadays, lots of patients have CGM's (Continuous Glucose Monitors) so they can easily correlate blood glucose level with diet.

Eating fat makes their blood glucose go up.

How come most people don't know that sat fat causes diabetes?

Most people focus on the hyperglycemia.

Hyperglycemia is easy to recognize.

It's the sat fat that starts it all.

Eat just one high fat meal, and insulin resistance starts a couple hours later.

Diabetic patients with CGM's (Continuous Glucose Monitors) will tell you that a high fat meal raises their blood sugar.

Sat fat alone can cause atherosclerosis as shown by the mummy studies; but atherosclerosis is much worse with added fructose, sodium, and PUFA's.

What about PUFA's?

I have not specifically read about the role of PUFA's in diabetes.

However, I have read that omega 6 PUFA's increase the risk of lipid peroxidation, and that can cause mitochondrial dysfunction, or even ferroptosis (cell death).

Sat fat causes mitochondrial dysfunction, that leads to insulin resistance. PUFA related mitochondrial dysfunction might worsen insulin resistance.

Omega 6 PUFA's are associated with inflammation, which is also bad.

What about omega 3 PUFA's?

There appears to be some association between omega 3 PUFA's and prostate cancer.

It's more difficult to purify omega 3's than is widely recognized.

Dietary supplementation might be associated with weight gain, and increased risk of atherosclerosis.

Omega 3's might have an immune suppressing effect, that is potentially detrimental in cancer patients.

What are you saying?

Stay away from junk food, animal food, and unnecessary extra stuff.

Eat the low fat vegan pyramid of starch, fruits, and vegetables.

This leads to an 80 : 10 : 10 — 80% carbohydrate : 10% protein : 10% fat — dietary intake.

People who do that are the healthiest people in the world.

How does saturated fat cause insulin resistance?

Saturated fat causes reversal of electron transport in the mitochondria.

Why does saturated fat cause reversal of electron transport?

Saturated fat is broken down by the "beta oxidation" pathway.

Beta oxidation is called that because the "beta" carbon gets oxidized to become a ketone.

One of the steps in beta oxidation is to form a double bond. This double bond forming step also produces an FADH2.

What is FADH2?

FADH2 is an electron carrier.

Where does FADH2 go?

FADH2 delivers electrons to coenzyme Q in the inner mitochondrial membrane.

Why is generation of FADH2 by forming a double bond in saturated fat during beta oxidation such a big deal?

Because coenzyme Q, and complex 3, get overwhelmed with electrons!!!!

What's coenzyme Q got to do with it?

Coenzyme Q normally delivers electrons to complex 3 in the inner mitochondrial membrane.

The inner mitochondrial membrane has electron transporters in this order: complex 1, complex 2, coenzyme Q, complex 3, cytochrome C, complex 4.

What happens when coenzyme Q and complex 3 get overwhelmed with electrons?

Then proton gradient between the inner mitochondrial matrix and the mitochondrial, intermembrane space goes too high; this causes shutdown of forward electron transport.

The sh_t hits the fan. Electron transport starts going backwards. Complex 1 makes superoxide anions.

Superoxide anions are a reactive oxygen species (ROS) that cause oxidative stress.

When electron transport gets backed up, what happens to the TCA cycle, and to glycolysis?

TCA cycle and glycolysis also get backed up.

What are the consequences of glycolysis getting backed up?

Harmful side pathways start to run, like for the production of AGE's (Advanced Glycation Endproducts) via Methyl GlyOxal (MGO).

MGO is a three carbon molecule — like propane —— with a ketone on the middle carbon —— and an aldehyde on the end carbon.

MGO reacts with proteins that have accessible sidechains of lysine and arginine, to form AGE's (Advanced Glycation Endproducts).

What about insulin resistance?

The saturated fat effect on the mitochondria causes the cell to sense "overnutrition."

The cell can't handle the saturated fat. The cell is suffering from "over nutrition." The cell certainly does NOT want any extra glucose coming into the cell.

The cell blocks the glut 4 transporter vesicles from going to the plasma membrane. Now glucose can't get into the cell.

Where is all this happening?

In skeletal muscle cells.

Why is insulin resistance in skeletal muscle a big deal?

Normally, 80-85% of postprandial glucose goes to skeletal muscle. Skeletal muscle is the perfect location for it, because any surplus is made into glycogen.

What happens when insulin resistance prevents the skeletal muscle from taking up glucose?

The glucose accumulates in the blood. High blood glucose is called HYPERglycemia.

What is the significance of hyperglycemia?

Skeletal muscle cells and adipose cells are dependent on insulin, and glut 4 transporters for uptake of glucose.

But some other cells in the body are not dependent on insulin, and glut 4 transporters.

What cells are not dependent on glut 4 transporters?

Endothelial cells are not dependent on insulin, and glut 4. With hyperglycemia, endothelial cells **TAKE UP TOO MUCH GLUCOSE**, and this causes microvascular disease.

Microvascular disease leads to atherosclerosis, arterial occlusion, myocardial infarction, and stroke.

Kidney cells are not dependent on glut 4. With hyperglycemia, kidney cells take up too much glucose, and this causes diabetic nephropathy.

Diabetic nephropathy causes kidney failure that leads to a progressive decline in health, and then death.

Peripheral nerves are not dependent on glut 4. With hyperglycemia, peripheral nerves take up too much glucose, and this causes peripheral neuropathy.

Peripheral neuropathy leads to loss of sensation in the foot, which leads to neuropathic arthropathy, also called Charcot joints.

Why is all this happening?

Because skeletal muscle cells are not good at controlling uptake of saturated fat!!!   And the person eats too much fat!

Why are skeletal muscle cells not good at controlling uptake of saturated fat?

Because humans are NOT made to eat saturated fat in large, daily quantities!!!

Are you saying that humans are not designed to eat meat?

Yes. Of course, humans can handle meat in small, occasional amounts, but when they eat meat in large amounts, on a daily basis, they become sick in middle age, or sooner.

What about the rest of the body?

If skeletal muscles are not designed to handle a high fat diet, then it makes sense that other parts of the body are also not designed for high fat diet.

The gut is not; sat fat causes leaky gut.

Blood is not; sat fat causes elevated LDL and resultant rouleaux formation of RBC's.

What are the other problems with hyperglycemia?

Glucose in the blood is almost entirely in the D ring form, or the L ring form; with ring forms being like a Haworth projection.

A tiny amount of glucose is in the linear form; with linear forms being like a Fischer projection.

Glucose in the linear form is an aldehyde, and relatively reactive.

Glucose in linear form can nonenzymatically bind to proteins, and this is called "glycation."

Linear glucose typically binds to lysine side chains of proteins. The initial binding might be reversible, but after the bond undergoes an Amadori rearrangement, it becomes essentially irreversible.

LDL cholesterol can also become glycated to become LDL-AGE. LDL-AGE can also bind R-AGE receptors.
These products of glycation are called "AGE's" (Advanced Glycation Endproducts).

101

How come you always write about diabetes prevention, and hardly ever about treatment?

Because, my goal is to prevent diabetes.

I'm a diagnostic-interventional-neuro radiologist, and a nutrition nerd.

I don't have diabetes. I don't actually treat diabetes patients.

I do see the complications of diabetes, all day long, every day. Diabetes is the highway to health hell.

Diabetes is the express route to myocardial infarction, stroke, foot amputation, kidney failure, blindness, and Alzheimer disease.

Diabetes is associated with Alzheimer's?

Yes. Alzheimer's disease is called type 3 diabetes.

Alzheimer's disease is also associated with increased aluminum, iron, and copper intake. One could say that Alzheimer's is "heavy metal diabetes."

How is Alzheimer's associated with diabetes?

The enzyme that removes insulin from the blood is called Insulino-lysin. Insulino-lysin also is needed to remove beta amyloid plaques from the brain.

High blood insulin levels deplete insulino-lysin.

Important brain cells have glut 4 transporters, and these suffer from relative hypoglycemia when there is insulin resistance.

High fat diets lead to high blood cholesterol levels. Animal protein also causes increased blood cholesterol. Fructose in processed foods causes high blood cholesterol.

High blood cholesterol is associated with increased risk of Alzheimer's,

102

especially in patients with abnormal cholesterol transport in the brain with the bad Apo E's.

Do you have any advice for people who already have type 2 diabetes?

Everything I've read screams that they should become 100%, low fat, low salt, whole food, plant based VEGANS!!

Avoiding meat completely will increase "carbohydrate tolerance."

This low fat vegan diet optimizes insulin sensitivity, optimizes energy levels, and minimizes complications.

Type 2 diabetics should eat more starch, fruits, and vegetables, and become 100% vegans.

What's new about diabetes since your last book?

In the past, **I underestimated the benefits of fruits.** Reading about vitamin C renewed my interest in eating more fruit.

Then I read that humans evolved color vision so they could recognize when fruit was ripe.

If we "evolved" color vision to help us eat fruits, then it seems likely that eating fruits is important for our health.

People probably ate LOTS of fruit, before they had fire, which enabled them to cook starch. People probably ate LOTS of fruit, before the agricultural expansion, about 10,000 years ago.

What else is good about fruits?

Fruits have a surprisingly large amount of fiber. Fiber is your friend.

One serving of fruits has 4 grams of fiber, the same as oatmeal!

People eat way too much protein.

Fruits have much less protein than oatmeal and beans!

What about the benefit of fruits for the kidneys?

When you lower your protein intake, you lower the workload of your kidneys.

What about alkalinity?

Fruits are more alkaline than grains!

The kidney has to manage dietary acid, like that from eating meat, with its heavy load of methionine. When you eat alkaline foods like fruits, you decrease the workload of your kidneys.

What about sodium?

Sodium is a vasoconstrictor, which is bad.

Fruits are low in sodium. If a person is an athlete, and sweats a lot, they will lose sodium in the sweat, and thus have an increased need for dietary sodium.

What about phosphate?

In general, dietary phosphate is something to be avoided.

Processed foods are the worst, and tend to lead to the absorption of lots of phosphate.

Meat is the second worst, and tend to lead to absorption of moderate amounts of phosphate.

Plant foods lead to the lowest amount of phosphate absorption.

What's the bottom line on fruits?

Most people should be eating more fruits.

Fruits are the second biggest level — (after starch) — on the low fat, vegan, dietary food pyramid (see preface).

What are the blood tests for diabetes?

Normal hemoglobin A1c is 5.5 or less.
Prediabetes is 5.6-6.4.
Diabetes is 6.5 and up.

Normal fasting blood sugar is 100 or less.
Prediabetes is 100-125.
Diabetes is > 125.

Should I walk when eating?

If others are around, it is nice to talk during meals.

If alone, it's good to walk during meals.

Walking during meals, or immediately after can lower postprandial blood glucose by up to 50%.

I always walk, and listen to audiobooks when eating, and yesterday, some salad spilled on the floor.

Grandma barked at me, "There's salad all over the floor — (a big exaggeration) — Why can't you sit down when you eat; like a normal person?"

Me, "To be *normal*, means to be fat. I want to be skinny."

If someone has diabetes, what should they read?

A good place to start is "Mastering Diabetes" by Cyrus Wombatta, and Bobby Bigpoo.

Those guys both have type 1 diabetes, and they are very smart, and they are experts in the vegan diet.

They both are largely "fruitarian" in their dietary approach.

Once they started eating lots of fruits, their insulin sensitivity improved, and so did their energy levels.

My other book "How to reduce risk of cancer and chronic disease" has much more coverage of the biochemistry and pathophysiology of diabetes.

Chapter 9

Kidneys, and rice

What does the kidney do?

Excretes protein waste called "nitrogen."

Balances blood pH, which mostly means correcting the acidosis induced by animal protein.

Do we need both kidneys?

No. A healthy person who donates a kidney, will still have "normal" renal function on lab tests; even though they now have only 50% of their previous renal function.

This has profound implications.

What is the significance of having a plasma creatinine of 1.5 (normal is 1.2 or less)?

It means that the patient has lost about 60% of their renal function. That's bad!

How is chronic kidney disease (CKD) categorized?

GFR means Glomerular Filtration Rate. GFR is the filtration rate of the kidneys, and higher is better.

Stages of chronic kidney disease:

1. Kidney injury, but normal GFR > 75.
2. GFR 60-75.
3. GFR 30-60.
4. GFR 15-29.
5. GFR < 15 (usually requires dialysis).

Can renal failure be reversed by a low protein diet?

It depends on the severity of kidney failure.

The more severe the kidney failure, the tighter the kidney's "budget" for nitrogen excretion.

In order for BUN (blood urea nitrogen) levels to drop down to normal, the dietary nitrogen intake, must be less than the kidneys excretion rate.

It depends on the cause of kidney failure. A one time insult, that has passed, can yield a stable situation.

If there is an ongoing hypertension, diabetes, or autoimmune disease, then that also has to be treated.

It depends on the type of protein.

What are the different types of protein?

There are two main types of protein.

Plant protein is good for kidneys in small to moderate amounts.

Animal protein is bad for kidneys. Protein supplements are super bad for kidneys.

Why is animal protein bad for kidneys?

Because animal protein comes packaged with additional nitrogen in the form of creatine and creatinine.

Because animal protein is ACIDIC.

Why is animal protein acidic?

Because animal protein has a lot more methionine than does plant protein.

Methionine degradation releases sulfur, which gets converted into sulfuric acid.

Sulfuric acid causes metabolic acidosis.

How does the body handle this metabolic acidosis?

To help control meat acid, the kidney produces ammonia which is a base.

In addition, to help control meat acid, the body leaches calcium carbonate from the bones to buffer the pH.

This calcium is then voided into the urine.

Wait a second. **Are you saying that meat causes osteoporosis?**

Yes.

"Extraordinary claims require extraordinary evidence."
                              - Pierre Laplace, French mathemagician.

Osteoporosis doesn't happen overnight; it usually takes about 50 or more years to become symptomatic.

The animal protein also increases ILGF (Insulin Like Growth Factor) which slightly increases bone mass. The net effect is ongoing, mild, calcium-bone loss.

So what? Why should anyone care about peeing out a little calcium?

Some of that calcium precipitates in the kidney tubules. Kidney tubule blockage by calcium precipitate reduces kidney function.

Calcium precipitate gradually builds up to form kidney stones. Kidney stones can be VERY painful. My father had a kidney stone, and he said it was like being kicked by a horse.

Have you ever seen a urologist's cystoscope?

109

Cystoscopes are about the diameter of your thumb, one centimeter.

The urologist pushes the cystoscope through the urethra, and into the urinary bladder, so that he can fish out the stones.

It's much better to prevent kidney stones, than to have to endure that.

How does one prevent kidney stones?

Don't eat **meat** – so you avoid calciuria.

Avoid **sodium** – excess sodium causes calciuria.

Minimize **caffeine** – becauses increases urinary calcium excretion.

Minimize intake of processed food **fructose**, because the increased urate production is associated with increased risk of kidney stones.

Avoid excess **dehydration**, but don't go drinking excess water; a lot of people drink large amounts of UNFILTERED water, and one can have side effects from that.

Be careful with bottled water, because almost all brands do NOT provide any nutritional information; they really should tell you the TDS, the pH, sodium, fluoride, aluminum, method of filtration.

Why do low protein diets sometimes fail to slow the progression of kidney failure?

One reason is that the person does not distinguish between animal protein, and plant protein.

Animal protein is a problem for the kidneys, because it is **acidic**.

The animal protein acid load creates increased work for the kidney.

Animal protein comes "packaged" with additional nitrogen in the form of creatine, and creatinine.

Animal foods lack antioxidants.

When a person eats a lot of animal protein, the kidney goes into "HYPERFILTRATION" mode.

What is hyperfiltration mode?

Hyperfiltration is when the kidney maximizes its filtration rate by increasing it's own blood pressure — in the kidney — in response to a heavy workload.

Chronic, high meat, acid loads, with resultant hyperfiltration, can lead to "exhaustion" of the kidney, and subsequent kidney failure.

Is acid load the only problem with meat?

It's worse than that. Meat is also associated with leaky gut.

Leaky gut is thought to be one of the most common causes of autoimmune disease.

Are leaky gut, excess protein, and acid load, the only problems with meat?

Meat is worse than that.

Meat contains a lot of saturated fat. The saturated fat causes elevated LDL cholesterol.

Red blood cells (RBC's) have a "zeta potential." The zeta potential is produced by sialic acid residues on the glycocalyx of the RBC plasma membrane.

What is a zeta potential?

RBC's have a net negative charge that repels other RBC's. The good thing about the zeta potential is that it prevents RBC's from sticking together.

The purpose of the zeta potential is to prevent RBC's from clotting.

What is the relationship between RBC zeta potential and LDL cholesterol?

The LDL cholesterol overcomes the zeta potential, and causes RBC's to stick together like a stack of coins, and this is called "rouleaux" formation.

Rouleaux means "stack of coins."

What is the significance of RBC rouleaux?

RBC rouleaux makes the blood thick, like a milkshake, instead of like water.

Thick blood requires the heart to generate increased pumping pressure. Increased pumping pressure means hypertension.

Hypertension causes atherosclerosis. Atherosclerosis blocks the renal arteries. Atherosclerosis gradually causes kidney failure.

And it's worse than that. The rouleaux formation itself, can plug up capillaries, and cause tissue hypoxia.

An article by Kuo showed that a high saturated fat meal can cause a 20% drop in arterial PO_2.

How come hardly anyone knows about that?

Because the hemoglobin – oxygen dissociation curve is relatively FLAT at the top.

We've got a lot of reserve, so that we can deliver more oxygen during vigorous exertion; so a healthy person doesn't notice the 20% drop in PO_2.

Okay, okay, I get it. Meat is bad for kidneys because of leaky gut, acidosis, kidney stones, atherosclerosis, and hypoxia.

Can a person with mild, kidney failure just eat a low protein, plant diet, and then expect great results?

That sounds like a good start, but there is more to know.

They must lower their protein intake a lot.

Who was Walter Kempner?

The great Dr Walter Kempner (1903-1997) was the metabolic wizard of his time, 1940-1992.

Who did Kempner train with?

Walter Kempner, like Hans Krebs, had trained with Otto Waarburg.

Waarburg, Krebs, and Kempner are three of the most famous biochemistry-nutrition experts of the 1900's.

How did Kempner's knowledge of mitochondria help him as a doctor?

Kempner was acutely aware of the effect of hypoxia on a cell.

When a cell is hypoxic, it cannot produce energy from electron transport-oxidative phosphorylation.

Saturated fat and sodium can cause hypoxia of kidney cells.

What was Kempner's great insight about kidneys?

Kempner had noticed that a drop in kidney function was sometimes reversible.

Kempner reasoned that the reversibility might be due to a reversal of hypoxia.

- **When salt and saturated fat are reduced,**

- **the kidney gets more oxygen,**

- **and is capable of performing more work.**

When dietary protein is reduced, the kidney's nitrogen excretion workload is decreased.

When animal protein is avoided, then acidosis is avoided, and the kidney's acid balancing workload is decreased.

When the kidney's functional capacity is higher than its workload, then blood tests for BUN and creatinine start improving!!!

What were the macronutrient numbers for the Kempner diet?

Kempner had noticed that rice eating populations were relatively healthy.

Kempner put his patients on a 90 : 5 : 5 diet.

That's 90% carbohydrate, 5% protein, and 5% fat.

Kempner often increased the percentage of carbohydrates to 95%!!!

Isn't Kempner also the guy who whipped his patients?

Yes. Kempner had a few patients that when they failed to comply with the rice diet, he whipped them.

Was Kempner a medical genius?

Yes.

Dr Kempner was a genius.

Was Kempner a charismatic?

Yes. I've seen the photos. Kempner was often surrounded by women. He had a Rasputin like charisma.

I call it the "duck, duck, duck, goose!" method.

Rasputin was "religion, religion, religion, goose!"

Kempner was "rice, rice, rice, goose!"

How come nothin like that ever happens to me?

Kempner became a multimillionaire, and he helped his secretaries to buy houses, and his female assistants traveled with him.

Sounds like a great setup for polygamy.

I wish I knew about Kempner when I was younger. I could have had a harem, instead of a wife who bosses me around. I could've been a contender.

How many patients did Kempner treat?

Kempner treated **over 18 thousand patients** with the rice diet. Kempner published his methods and results in medical journals.

People from all over the world — including many rich and famous persons — traveled to Durham to be treated by Dr. Kempner.

Kempner's rice diet clinic was so popular, that it kept expanding into the local neighborhood, with bed and breakfast places, that were called "rice houses."

Durham became known as the best "diet city" in the world.

What kind of results did Kempner see?

Kempner often saw dramatic results with his patients.

Many patient made dramatic improvements in blood pressure, body weight, and kidney function.

How did Kempner follow his patients?

Kempner followed his patients with:

Chest x-rays that sometimes showed **normalization** of heart size.

Retinal photographs, that sometimes showed **reversal of disease**.

EKG's that sometimes showed **improvement**.

Body weight, blood pressure, renal function, and cholesterol which often showed **improvement**.

John McDougall MD, who is considered by many to be the best nutrition doctor in the world, said that Walter Kempner was one of his heroes.

Kempner's patients got all of their calories from plant foods and sugar.

Most of their calories were from **WHITE RICE**, and Kempner's diet was called the "Rice" diet.

Kempner also allowed the patients to eat **fruits**, and to drink **fruit juice** and **sugar water**.

Kempner preferred fruit juice over water, because fruit juice is alkaline, and he thought this helped the body to buffer acidosis.

Kempner's patients typically travelled to Durham, North Carolina, and were under his direct supervision for at least 2 weeks, and often 2 months or more.

Even after they went home, they had frequent urine and blood tests, so that Kempner could make sure everything was going well.

Is that all there is to it? Just eat tons of rice, and fruits, and avoid animal foods?

There's more to it than that.

One must also minimize sodium!

What's sodium got to do with it?

Sodium is a potent vasoconstrictor, because sodium inhibits endothelial nitric oxide.

What is normal sodium dietary intake?

The Yanomamo in South America who eat their traditional plant based diet, eat about 150-200 mg of sodium per day.

Dr. Kempner restricted his patients to **150 mg of SODIUM** per day.

Aren't "low" sodium diets usually around 2,000 mg per day?

Yes. They are typically 10x higher than the Yanomamo or Kempner approach.

Okay, so now we've got a plan, right?

Low fat plants, like rice, and low sodium. Is that all one needs to know?

It depends on the degree of kidney failure. When kidney failure becomes severe, then the patient might also have to restrict potassium intake.

Kidney failure patients also need to avoid excess phosphate intake.

The kidneys are kind of complicated.

Mild kidney failure patients, which is the majority, can start improving their health by changing to a low fat, low salt, vegan diet. Mild kidney failure patients are outpatients, and they can be managed by primary care doctors.

Moderate and severe kidney failure patients should be referred to a kidney specialist, called a nephrologist.

Why are nephrologists the worst doctors to date?

They are always getting pissed off!

How to protect kidneys:

- **Low fat** diet to avoid hypertension, atherosclerosis, and hypoxia.

- **Low sodium** to avoid hypertension, atherosclerosis, and hypoxia.

- **Low** in processed **fructose** — like sugary drinks — to avoid uric acid and LDL cholesterol related hypertension, atherosclerosis, and hypoxia.

- **No animal foods** to avoid leaky gut, and acidosis.

- **No processed foods** to avoid sodium, oils, and phosphates.

- **100% plant foods**, but limit beans, because beans are high in protein.

- 100% plant foods, but limit grains, because grains are slightly acidic.

- Plant foods tend to be alkaline, especially fruits and vegetables, so they lower the workload of the kidneys.

- Plant foods are low in fat and cholesterol, so they help avoid hypertension, diabetes, and atherosclerosis.

- Plant foods are high in antioxidants.

- Plant foods have fiber, so they help to prevent leaky gut.

- Plant foods are low in sodium. There is ZERO sodium in blueberries, oatmeal, quinoa.

Why do kidney failure patients get so much arterial calcification?

Kidney failure patients often have proteinuria, loss of protein in the urine.

Proteinuria is associated with lowering of a protein called "Fetuin-A."

What is Fetuin-A?

Fetuin A is made by the liver, and helps prevent arterial calcification.

Chronic kidney disease with metabolic acidosis tends to lead to proteinuria, and decreased Fetuin-A.

Low protein, low fat, plant based diet helps prevent kidney failure, and proteinuria.

What else helps prevent arterial calcification?

Avoid excess dietary calcium.

Avoid excess dietary phosphorus, which means avoiding processed foods, and meat.

Avoiding atherosclerosis helps prevent arterial calcification.

Maintaining adequate magnesium levels helps prevent arterial calcification.

Why do kidney failure patients develop anemia?

In part because the kidney is less able to make erythropoietin.

I think it's also in part due to high blood viscosity. The body is able to monitor blood viscosity.

I learned this from reading Gregory Sloop MD who said that, **"ANEMIA OF CHRONIC DISEASE" IS OFTEN A PHYSIOLOGIC RESPONSE**

High blood viscosity decreases tissue perfusion. Paradoxically, lowering the hematocrit, can sometimes improve tissue "perfusion," because a lowered hematocrit means lower blood viscosity.

When the cause of high blood viscosity — like dietary saturated fat or leaky gut or an infection — is removed, the hemoglobin might return to normal.

Are there any problems with a plant based diet for kidney failure patients?

Be careful with beans, because they contain a lot of protein.

Be careful with brown rice, and oats, because they have a slightly high acid load.

When kidney failure gets more severe, there is increased risk of problems with hyperkalemia (high potassium).

The worse the level of kidney failure, the more closely the patient needs to be monitored by a physician.

Very sweet fruits, like bananas, can sometimes cause rebound hypoglycemia.

Unusual fruits like strawberries, which have complex shapes, that make it difficult to rinse them off, should only be eaten when organic.

Which patients were the most complicated for Kempner to treat?

The kidney failure patients. With kidney failure, one has to pay attention to phosphorus, albumin, and potassium, as well as animal protein, and saturated fat.

With weight loss, and hypertension patients who have good kidneys, management is easier.

Chapter 10

Female problems and Estrogen

Normal estrogen levels are a blessing.

High estrogen levels are a curse.

What problems are caused by (or associated with) high estrogen levels?

- Dysfunctional uterine bleeding with long periods.

- Menstrual cramps.

- PMS.

- Endometriosis.

- Morning sickness of pregnancy.

- Postpartum depression.

- Obesity.

- Fibroids.

- Adenomyosis of the uterus = endometrial-glandular tissue in the myometrial -muscle layer of the uterus.

- Increased risk autoimmune diseases.

- Increased risk post menopausal hot flashes.

- Increased benign breast masses, like fibrocystic disease.

- Increased risk breast cancer.

- Increased risk endometrial cancer.

Why do so many woman have high estrogen levels?

- Eating meat.

    - Because the liver conjugates estrogen with another chemical, and then excretes it into the bile.

    - Normally, women poop out their extra estrogen.

    - Meat changes gut bacteria.

    - Meat based gut bacteria have the enzyme "glucoronidase" to deconjugate estrogen.

    - This deconjugated estrogen is then reabsorbed from the gut, back into the blood.

- Drinking whole milk.

    - Nowadays, the milk cow is usually engineered to produce milk while it's pregnant.

    - Pregnant cows have very high estrogen levels.

    - Pregnant cow, extra estrogen, gets into the milk.

- Drinking water that contains estrogens.

    - Municipal water filtration often does not remove estrogens well;

    - like EE2 (Ethinyl Estradiol of birth control pills) and atrazine (herbicide).

    - Yes. Your tap water might contain EE2, and atrazine.

- Storing drinks in BPA, or other estrogenic containers.

- Just because the container says, "no BPA," it might be a BPA substitute like BPS, which is still estrogenic.

- Watch out for cans. The lining of cans often is made with BPA.

- Cosmetic skin products with estrogenic preservatives like the parabens.

- Soaps and shampoos with estrogen. I use the safest of newborn baby shampoos, and it still contains an estrogenic.

- Laundry detergents with estrogen.

  - A typical detergent is nonoxynol-9, an estrogen.

  - The plastic container is often made out of BPA, and pthalates, which are both estrogenic.

  - That's three estrogens on your "clean" clothes.

  - All day long, these clothes contact your skin, and estrogen is absorbed through your skin, and into your blood.

What else can a woman do to normalize her estrogen levels?

- Avoid meat and milk.

- Do not put cosmetic products on her skin; especially avoid aluminum deodorant.

  - We greet each other by saying, "Hello."

  - We do not sniff each other's armpits.

  - If you are a low IQ, wimpy conformist who insists on wearing deodorant, then at least do NOT shave your pits.

- Shaving increases transdermal absorption.

- Wash clothes without detergent. Just run the washer and dryer longer and hotter.

- Store beverages in glass.

- Obtain a carbon filter, or reverse osmosis filter for water.

What's the key concept for understanding estrogen disrupting chemicals (EDC's)?

Estrogen, the hormone, for millions of years, in the animal kingdom, had no competition.

Estradiol is the main form of estrogen. The active part of the estradiol molecule is the "phenol group."

A phenol group is a hydroxy group attached to a benzene. The benzene ring is also called an aromatic ring because it gives off an "aroma."

Benzene rings are cyclohexanes with three double bonds that resonate; this resonance confers super stability; this stuff can sit on a shelf for years, and remain unchanged.

The hydroxy group (phenol group) confers antimicrobial activity.

Do you get it?

Estrogenic chemicals, like parabenzoic acid, are the **PERFECT PRESERVATIVE**; long shelf life, and antimicrobial.

That's why EDC's (Estrogen Disrupting Chemicals) are almost always put into skin care products.

That's why I recommend to **avoid all skin care products**.

What should people do with their cosmetic products?

In the 1490's Girolamo Savanarola called for a **BONFIRE OF THE VANITIES**.

It is time to call for a bonfire of cosmetic vanities.

If women want to burn their bras too, men won't complain.

Just kidding. You don't need to burn your cosmetics — that would create toxic smoke — but you should throw most of that junk into the garbage.

Why do these chemicals have an estrogenic effect?

The estrogen receptor simply recognizes the "phenol group" component of the molecule for activation. The estrogen receptor doesn't care much what is attached to the phenol group.

During the millions of years during which the estrogen receptor was "evolving," these other chemicals did not exist.

The estrogen receptor is a bit of a "slut." Just show her a phenol group, and she will open up, and hydrogen bond with it, and get activated.

What happens when the estrogen receptor gets activated?

Estrogen causes proliferation of breast cells, and endometrial cells.

Excess estrogen, and EDC's can lead to excess proliferation of breast, and endometrial cells, with resultant cancer.

Where can one learn more about estrogen biochemistry, and disease avoidance?

In my other book, "How to prevent cancer and chronic disease," I go into much more detail about estrogen physiology, and which products, and preservatives are estrogenic.

125

What about PCOS?

PCOS is Poly Cystic Ovary Syndrome. PCOS has several causes: genetic vulnerability, obesity, diabetes, and potentially elevated intracranial pressure (as it relates to CSF pressure theory).

Obesity and diabetes are asssociated with a decrease in steroid hormone binding globulin (SHBG).

Normally, SHBG binds to androgens and estrogens in the blood. When blood levels of SHBG are lowered, then there is more "free" estrogen and androgen going around causing problems.

What's the benefit of low fat, low salt, vegan diet for PCOS?

Optimizes body weight, so that obesity goes away, and diabetes might go away, and SHBG levels increase.

Avoiding exogenous estrogenics like BPA, aluminum, nonoxynol 9, parabens and so on, can help for treatment of PCOS.

Only eat organic foods. Nonorganic food is more likely to have residues from estrogenic herbicides like atrazine.

Here's a little verse to keep it terse:

- Estrogenics make you fat and SICK.

- They hide in lotion and PLASTIC.
- Go through your skin like MAGIC.

- Feminization of frogs and FISHES,
- Messes up her cycle.
- Turns Betties into BITCHES.

- Woman got no baby.
- Man got no D_CK.

- Molecular memory, it's real SLICK.
- Autoimmune and ALLERGIC.

- Now we know their little TRICK,
- We gonna avoid them real QUICK.

The inspiration for the above poem was the lovely childhood rhyme I learned in 7th grade when the girls were skipping rope and singing:

- "Ding, dong, you're momma don'na wear no drawers.

- I saw her when she took'em off.

- She laid them on the table.

- Them fruits ain't got no flava."

Chapter 11

Cancer

What are the three phases of cancer?

#1. **Initiation** = DNA damage = **mutation** = caused by a carcinogen = turns off cell growth regulation.

Some cancer is thought caused by random mutation, otherwise known as bad luck; but just because a cancer is present, that doesn't mean it will grow.

The mutation can be activation of an "oncogene," which means a gene capable of causing cancer;

or a mutation that turns off a "tumor suppressor gene," which means a gene that normally suppresses cancer.

Initiation is emphasized by the **"mutation theory of cancer."**

DNA gets damaged all the time, and the cell is usually good at repairing it.

Genetic vulnerabilities are associated with less ability to repair DNA, and these are emphasized with **"genetic, or family history, theories of cancer."**

#2. **Promotion** = something causes abnormal growth of a cancer cell.

Promotion is emphasized by **"metabolic theory of cancer."**

In reality, cancer causation and growth is a **combination of 1, genetic vulnerabilities, 2. carcinogens inducing mutation, and 3. metabolism.**

#3. **Metastasis** = distant spread of tumor.

Brain and lung metastases often cause death.

People usually don't die from the original primary tumor; they usually die from the metastases.

Women do not die from the tumor in their breast; They die from metastasis.

What are the three main pathways to cancer?

Genetic, mutation, and metabolic. Genetic causes are rare.

Cancer causation is usually a combination of mutation, and abnormal metabolism.

Why do some cells become cancerous?

A normal cell can become "cancerous" when its **"growth control" DNA** is damaged and not repaired.

Cancer growth is suppressed by **tumor suppressor genes,** which include genes **for DNA repair.**

Cancer cells tend to undergo **"aerobic-anaerobic" glycolysis** = burning glucose for energy without using the mitochondria.

The mitochondrial electron transport system is **oxygen** dependent for energy production.

What is the Waarburg effect?

Cancer cells running on glycolysis burn through a lot of glucose, and this is called the Waarburg effect.

"The prime cause of cancer is the replacement of normal oxygen respiration in cells by fermentation [anaerobic glycolysis]."

- Otto Waarburg, Nobel prize winner 1931.

What Otto is saying is that healthy cells **fully** metabolize glucose in healthy mitochondria by transferring electrons to **oxygen**;

Cancer cells only **partially** metabolize glucose;

because cancer cells have **damaged mitochondria.**

Clinical oncologists, surgical oncologists, and radiation therapists are experts on the mutation component of cancer.

This guides choice of chemotherapy, surgery, and radiation therapy.

To also help yourself, you should learn about the benefits of:

- Stress reduction.
- Sleep optimization.
- Simplifying your life so you have time for exercise and sleep.
- Eating low fat vegan to improve the metabolic component of cancer.

You choose what you eat, and that might have a big effect on your cancer rate of growth, according to the research of Ornish, Campbell, Heidrich, McDougall, Pedersen, and others.

What is cancer milieu?

Milieu is the local environment of cancer cells.

Cancer milieu has what key characteristics?

Otto Waarburg noted that different types of cancer tend to produce increased **lactic acid**.

The cancer cells secrete lactic acid into the extracellular matrix.

The immune system normally can remove cancer cells.

Lactic acid **IMPAIRS THE IMMUNE SYSTEM** by blocking activation of CD8+ T and NK cells.

Running on glycolysis enables cancer cells to keep growing in low oxygen conditions.

Cancer cell ability to grow in low oxygen conditions enables cancer cells to **out proliferate the surrounding cells**.

This glycolysis dependent behavior led to the recognition that cancer cells tend to have **MITOCHONDRIAL DYSFUNCTION.**

Cancer cell replication and growth is **"promoted"** by ongoing exposure to conditions that favor cancer growth.

Cancer cells tend to develop a localized **hypoxic, acidotic milieu.**

Hypoxic, acidotic milieu.

Hypoxic, acidotic milieu.

Normal cells do not function well in a hypoxic, acidotic milieu.

A hypoxic, acidotic milieu enables cancer cells to outgrow neighboring cells.

What are tumor promoters?

Things that favor cancer growth.

The common tumor promoters are:

- **Alcohol,**
- **Tobacco,**
- **Animal protein,**
- **Animal fat,**
- **Oils,**
- **Estrogenics**

What's the significance of tumor promoters?

Everyone has been exposed to carcinogens. Everyone has some DNA mutations.

Almost all of these will be of no significance.

You certainly should avoid carcinogens when you can, but it is more important to **FOCUS ON AVOIDING TUMOR PROMOTERS.**

It usually takes multiple decades for a cancer to become clinically relevant.

Our bodies are GREAT at repairing damaged DNA.

The smart move is to avoid tumor promoters so that a mutant cell never gets activated to become a clinically relevant cancer.

What is an easy way to remember the common tumor promoters?

Anything that's bad for your arteries probably increases the risk of cancer.

What's good for the heart is good for the brain, and helps prevent cancer.

What can a person do to try to decrease the risk of cancer growth?

You want to promote a well oxygenated, normal pH milieu!

Vegan diet prevents rouleaux, and hypertension, and atherosclerosis, and therefore tends to increase **oxygen** delivery to tissues.

Vegan diet is **alkaline** compared to meat diet. Just eat vegan foods. Do not go doing other crazy stuff about alkalinity. Your blood has to maintain a pH of around 7.4.

The key point is the **LOCAL** milieu of the cancer.

What about reducing animal protein?

Vegan diet is low in the essential amino acids called leucine and methionine.

Cancer needs lots of leucine and methionine for making proteins, and replicating DNA.

Cancer needs lots of nitrogen for making proteins and replicating DNA.

T Colin Campbell's research showed that when animal protein gets over 10% of calories, there is a big increase in cancer risk.

Cancer especially ramps up metabolism of glutamine which is a "conditionally" essential amino acid.

Plant diets help to deprive cancer of the leucine and methionine that cancer wants. Vegan diet reduces the risk of getting cancer.

The average person "wants" to eat more animal protein. A well informed person fears animal protein, and avoids it.

What about prostate cancer?

Prostate cancer is hormonal, similar to breast cancer; increased risk with estrogenic chemicals.

It ain't the young guys with high testosterone who get prostate cancer. It's the old guys with low testosterone who get prostate cancer.

Check out the research of Dr. Ornish on diet and PSA.

What causes mitochondrial dysfunction?

- **Hypoxia**.

    - Hypoxia causes dysfunction because oxygen is needed to serve as the ultimate electron acceptor in electron transport.
    - Otto Waarburg showed in the 1920's that when cells are hypoxic, they sometimes become cancerous.

- **Saturated fat.**

    - Saturated fat, beta-oxidation yields the maximum number of FADH2 electron carriers, and this tends to overwhelm electron transport between coenzyme Q and complex 3.
    - Saturated fat causes reversal of electron transport, and increased production of ROS.

- **Intracellular hyperglycemia.**

    - Some cells are not glut 4 (insulin dependent glucose type 4 transporter) dependent.
    - These cells take up glucose continuously, and in the

133

presence of hyperglycemia, can be flooded by glucose.
- This INTRAcellular HYPERglycemia can also overwhelm electron transport, and lead to it's reversal.
- INTRAcellular HYPERglycemia is typically caused by poorly controlled, insulin dependent diabetes.

- **PUFA's (PolyUnsaturated Fatty Acids)**

  - PUFA's are vulnerable to lipid peroxidation, especially in the setting of free-unliganded iron.
  - Lipid peroxidation can set off a chain reaction — like dominos — in mitochondrial membranes.
  - Mitochondrial membranes contain a lot of PUFA's.

- **Mitochondrial toxins,** like some pesticides. Pesticides tend to bioaccumulate in nonorganic meat.

In addition to hypoxia, saturated fat, intracellular hyperglycemia, and free iron, what else can generate a lot of ROS?

The enzyme, NADPH oxidase which is sometimes abbreviated Nox.

Nox can be "overactivated" by AGE's. AGE's are Advanced Glycation Endproducts.

Hyperglycemia (excess glucose in the blood caused by diabetes) can glycate proteins to form AGE's.

Hemoglobin A1-C is a blood test that indicates glycation.

AGE's can bind Receptors for AGE's that are called R-AGE receptors.

Binding of AGE's to R-AGE receptors causes activation of NADPH Oxidase, and generation of ROS, like superoxide anions.

What stimulates a cell to grow, and possibly proliferate?

- Insulin is anabolic.

- ILGF (Insulin Like Growth Factor) is anabolic.

- Estrogen stimulates cell proliferation in the breast, endometrium, and prostate.

- Leucine is a branched chain, amino acid that stimulates mTOR. MTOR is a nutrient sensing system, and a growth regulator.

- When mTOR senses that nutrients are widely available, it "tells" the cells to grow.

- MTOR overactivation is thought to contribute to growth in the majority of cancers.

- Methionine is an essential amino acid for cancer growth. Meat has much more methionine, than do plant foods.

What causes DNA mutations?

Carcinogen chemicals, tobacco smoke, alcohol, hypoxia, insulin resistance. Deficiencies of folate and vitamin B12.

Anything that increases oxidative stress, like PUFA's, and unliganded iron, can increase mutations. Oxidative stress means increased reactive oxygen species (ROS). ROS can cause mutations.

What is a proto-oncogene?

A proto-oncogene is a gene, that if mutated could cause cancer.

What is an oncogene?

An oncogene is a gene that is contributing to the cause of cancer.

What is p53?

P53 is a tumor suppressor gene because it helps for DNA repair.

- p53 is sometimes called "the guardian of the genome."
- p53 protein helps recognize double stranded DNA breaks.
- p53 then activates a pathway to repair the DNA.
- If the DNA cannot be repaired, then p53 signals for the cell go into apoptosis.
- Mutations in p53 cause increased risk of cancer.
- P53 mutation is the most common mutation in cancers.
- Benzpyrene, a carcinogen in cigarettes, binds the p53 gene, leading to cancer.

Things that decrease risk of cancer:

Vegan diet.

- No animal protein.

    - That's right! **ZERO** animal protein!

- Fish is not okay.

    - It's all animal muscle.
    - Animal muscle means animal protein, and saturated fat.
    - All animal muscle should be avoided.
    - Even if it's grass fed, it's still got animal protein and saturated fat.

- Even a small amount of animal protein can cause a big increase in risk of cancer.

- The graph of cancer frequency vs meat consumption is linear, about a 45 degree line, with about 1:1 correlation between meat intake, and cancer rate, and it goes through zero;

- there is no safe amount of meat, not associated with an increase risk of cancer.

- **Meat is unsafe "at any speed."**

- Even animal protein intakes as low as 3% of calories appear to be associated with increased risk of cancer.

- Therefore, you want ZERO, none, nada, not one bite, not one nanometer!

- Plant foods are super low in saturated fat.

- Plant foods have lots of **ANTIOXIDANTS** like vitamin C.

- Green vegetables like salad and broccoli, often increase **NITRIC OXIDE** and blood flow.

- Greens are **ALKALINE**, and thus help prevent acidosis.

AVOID ANIMAL PROTEIN.

- Animal protein causes increased blood cholesterol, and atherosclerosis. (That's not a misprint. Animal PROTEIN does cause increased cholesterol).
- Animal protein is a tumor promoter.
- Animal protein increases ILGF.
- Leucine is more common in animal protein.

    - Leucine activates mTOR, a nutrient sensing, growth regulator.

    - When large amounts of leucine are present, mTOR "senses" nutrients are widely available, and might increase cell growth and proliferation.

- Methionine is more common in animal protein.
    - Cancer cells want more methionine.

AVOID ANIMAL FAT.

- Animal fat means saturated fat.

137

- Animal fat increase is associated with increased risk of cancer.

- Populations that do not eat meat or oils, have an amazingly low incidence of breast cancer.

- The more animal fat a person eats, the higher their risk of cancer.

- In countries where people eat a lot of animal fat, there is a lot of colon cancer, breast cancer, and prostate cancer.

- Saturated fat causes RBC rouleaux, and tissue hypoxia.

- Saturated fat tends to cause mitochondrial dysfunction.

- Animal fat causes increased cholesterol level.

- Increased cholesterol is associated with increased risk of atherosclerosis and cancer.

- The chemical formula for cholesterol is $C_{27}H_{46}O$.

- High cholesterol can lead to increased production of a cholesterol metabolite called, **27-hydroxy-cholesterol.**

- Some cancers, like tamoxifen resistant breast cancer, sometimes feed on 27-hydroxy-cholesterol.

- The enzyme Cyp27-A1 converts cholesterol into 27-hydroxy cholesterol.

- 27 hydroxy-cholesterol can have an estrogenic, tumor promoting effect on breast cancer cells.

- Some speculate that 27 hydroxy-cholesterol can contribute to reactivation of breast cancer in some patients, such as those that are resistant to tamoxifen.

- 27-hydroxy-cholesterol appears to be a tumor promoter that might increase the risk of breast cancer metastases.

- The ideal cholesterol is TOTAL cholesterol always below 150.

- Note: this is **TOTAL** cholesterol below 150.

- Total cholesterol below 150 is the key therapeutic goal for preventing atherosclerosis, (which is another way of saying, increasing tissue oxygenation).

- If your total cholesterol is below 150, your LDL will be okay. However, if you want a number goal for LDL, then try to get it down to 60 mg/dl.

Eat starch to:

- Provide fiber, and prevent leaky gut; thus reduce inflammation.
- Provide fiber and promote gut flora that increases estrogen removal from the body by defecation.

Eat fruits and vegetables:

- High in antioxidants, like vitamin C, which protect DNA, and mitochondria.
- Lower blood viscosity, which improves blood flow, which prevents hypoxia.
- Alkaline to possibly decrease cancer related acidotic milieu.
- Low in methionine and leucine.
- Cruciferous vegetables are thought especially protective, like broccoli, and brussel sprouts.

Exercise.

- Exercise dramatically decreases risk of breast cancer; and the more the exercise, the more the risk reduction.
- 11 minutes of walking reduces risk by 20%. 4 hrs/week reduces risk by 40%. 5 or more hours per week reduces risk by about 60%.
- Kind of reminds you of triathletes like Ruth Heydrich.
- Everybody knows that walking contracts leg muscles which squeeze the veins, and this helps return blood to the heart.
- Everybody knows that the leg veins have valves to facilitate

unidirectional blood flow.
- But did you know that there's another system of "vessels with valves" in your legs; and throughout your body?

It's called the LYMPHATIC SYSTEM!!!

When you walk, you get your lymph to flow. When your lymph flows, your WBC's travel around the body to search for cancer cells, and remove them.

What are the other benefits of exercise?

- Walking helps your WBC's to do their job of protecting you.

    - Exercise increases nitric oxide vasodilator to open up arteries.

    - Exercise improves tissue perfusion.

    - Exercise improves physical appearance.

    - Exercise improves self esteem.

    - Exercise lowers stress levels.

Sleep at night.

At least one good social relationship.

- *Social support increases survival with breast cancer.*

Helping at least one other person on a routine basis.

    - Improves self esteem.

    - Lowers stress levels.

    - When you help others, you help yourself.

    - A mood booster because of reward neurotransmitters that approve of you doing things that will help you to maintain acceptance by the social group.

Love

- To be loved makes a person feel safe which lowers their stress levels.

- To love someone and try to help them gives a person a sense of purpose.

    - A sense of purpose lowers stress levels.

A purpose in life

- Energizes a person.

- Improves self esteem.

- Increased happiness.

Avoid things that increase cancer risk.

Carcinogens include:
- Benzopyrene in cigarette smoke.
- Heterocyclic amines in meat.
- Alcohol,
- Asbestos.
- Aflatoxin,
- Arsenic,
- Benzene,
- Dioxin.

Genetic vulnerabilities to cancer.

- BRCA1 and BRCA2 genes are involved in DNA repair.
- Women with defects in either the BRCA1 or BRCA2 genes have increased risk of breast cancer.

EDC's

EDC's increase risk of breast cancer, and that is covered in other chapters of this book.

Be careful what you put in your mouth; alcohol, mouthwash, toothpaste, tobacco can all be carcinogenic and/or estrogenic.

SEDENTARY

ALUMINUM

Armpit and breast lymphatics are connected.

Breast cancer (BC) is most common in the upper outer quadrant (UOQ).

UOQ BC has increased percentage wise in past century.

Theory is that armpit aluminum deodorant increases BC risk.

Aluminum is a "metalloestrogen" that can stimulate growth of BC.

BC risk is increased if a woman shaves first, before applying aluminum, because nicks in skin can increase absorption.

Humans are not dogs.

We don't greet each other by sniffing butts or armpits.

You don't need to wear deodorant!

EDC's (Estrogen Disrupting Chemicals) from other skin care products like sunscreen, and paraben preservatives, can increase risk of cancer.

ALCOHOL

Beverage alcohol is ethanol, C-C-OH. Ethanol is converted in liver to acetaldehyde, C-CH=O.

Acetaldehyde is thought to be carcinogenic and increase BC risk. Alcohol decreases immune function. Alcohol can lead to decreased thiamine, with resultant decreased cognitive function.

Alcohol can decrease folate, which can lead to impaired DNA synthesis, which leads to uracils being inserted into DNA, instead of Thymines, with resultant increased mutations.

Liver conversion of ethanol to acetaldehyde and acetate, C-C=O & O-generates NADPH which signals to store fats (instead of burn them) leading to fatty liver.

Alcohol effect on fat metabolism apparently is the reason that alcohol "stiffens" red blood cell (RBC) cell membranes.

Stiff RBC's means less flexible RBC's.

Less flexible RBC's means increased blood viscosity.

Increased blood viscosity means high blood pressure.

High blood pressure causes atherosclerosis.

Atherosclerosis causes tissue hypoxia.

Tissue hypoxia favors cancer cells.

Alcohol is a tumor promoter.

Increased alcohol causes increased risk of head and neck cancers.

Head and neck cancer cancers are bad cancers.

Head and neck cancer surgery routinely removes the tongue and the larynx (voicebox).

Alcohol also increases risk of esophageal cancer.

Esophageal cancer is a bad cancer.

The last thing in the world that I would want to do, is pour a tumor promoter, over my tongue, and larynx, and esophagus.

I do not drink alcohol.

Not one drop.

Breast cancer risk factors:

95% of breast cancer patients are over 40 years old when diagnosed. The median age of breast cancer diagnosis is 62 years old. Why is it that older women with "low" estrogen production, get breast cancer, instead of older women with "high" estrogen production?

Maybe because older women are fatter, and the fat tissue has the enzyme "aromatase," to make estrogen. Maybe it's because of the increased accumulation of estrogenic chemicals, and because their immune systems are weaker, and they have more atherosclerosis.

Anything that increases estrogen (unopposed).

- Obesity is the most probably the most important controllable risk factor.
- Early menarche.
- Late menopause.
- Nulliparity.
- Late age of childbearing.
- No breast feeding.
- Long term OCP's (oral contraceptive pills).
- Long term HRT (hormone replacement therapy).
- Estrogenic chemicals in deodorants, and other cosmetic products.
- Estrogenic chemicals in laundry detergents.
- Chemicals in processed food and meat like pesticides, herbicides, and food dyes as some of these are estrogenic.
- Drinking water that contains high levels of estrogenic chemicals.

Other general risk factors for cancer:

- High animal protein diet.
- High animal fat diet.
- Alcohol.
- Tobacco.
- Obesity.

- Diabetes.
- Sedentary.
- Silicone gel breast implants, especially if wrapped in polyurethane foam.
- Dark hair dyes with prolonged use.
- Electric blankets.
- Cleaning chemicals.
- Live near gas station or refinery.
- Lack of sleep.
- BRCA is a tumor suppressor gene that when mutated causes increased risk of breast cancer. 90-95% of breast cancer is not genetic. 87% of breast cancer patients do not have any first degree relatives with breast cancer. If an identical twin has breast cancer, her twin only has a 20% increase in risk of breast cancer; same as if her nontwin sister had breast cancer.

Read about cancer

- Read the work of T. Colin Campbell PhD, Kristi Funk MD, Dean Ornish MD, and Dr. John Kelly, and Ruth Heidrich PhD, and others.

- Consider join a support group so can talk to someone about life with cancer.

What is the connection between excess estrogen and cancer?

Elevated estrogen increases risk of breast cancer, endometrial cancer, and prostate cancer.

Persons who eat a lot of animal fat, tend to become fat themselves, which increases estrogen levels.

Eating **MEAT INCREASES ESTROGEN LEVELS** because meat causes a change in gut bacteria.

Normally, estrogen is conjugated in the liver, and then excreted in the stool.

Meat induced gut bacteria **cause DECONJUGATION of estrogen** so that it is reabsorbed back into the body.

This is called the enterohepatic circulation.

Meat related RE-absorption of estrogen causes increased blood levels of estrogen.

Meat eaters have higher blood levels of estrogen.

Plant eaters poop out their excess estrogen.

Fiber essentially PULLS ESTROGEN OUT OF YOUR BODY.

Yea!

Female meat eaters have increased breast carcinoma, and uterine fibroids.

Female vegetarians are less likely to get breast cancer.

Populations that eat a low fat vegan diet, have low rates of breast and prostate cancer.

Populations that eat moderate to high amounts of meat have high rates of breast and prostate cancer.

Does that mean it's okay to eat small amounts of meat?

No!

As cancer grows, it acquires more mutations, and becomes more aggressive, more malignant.

I've read about a lot of cancer patients who were in remission, and then they went back to old habits of eating meat, and oils, and salt, and their cancer came back, and killed them.

Some cancers have **OVEREXPRESSION OF RECEPTORS** for

growth factors which can lead to an amplified growth response.

Do not take a chance. My advice is do not take one bite of meat ever again in your life. And no oils.

My guess is that cancer cells can become **SENSITIZED** to growth factors, such that even small amounts of meat related tumor promoters might have a big effect.

There are times in life when you must move on to better things, and don't look back.

Lot's wife looked back, and she was turned into a pillar of salt.

Orpheus looked back, and Eurydice was dragged back into Hell.

How come older woman get more breast cancer even though they are postmenopausal with decreasing endogenous estrogen levels?

Older persons have weaker immune systems.

Older persons have accumulated lots of estrogenic chemicals from aluminum deodorant, skin moisturizers-sunscreen-colognes-perfumes, laundry detergent, and eating meat.

From what I've seen, women love to rub cosmetic "crap" on themselves. My mom used to do that, and she died of cancer.

My wife has about 55 cosmetic products that she rubs on herself. I told her that she is a stupid monkey playing with chemicals that she doesn't understand.

Wife: You don't understand. A woman would rub sh_t on her face, if she thought it would make her pretty.

Me: That's a big assumption, to think this stuff is going to make you prettier. These magic creams are not going to help you to lose weight.

147

Wife: I'm not fat. I'm just chubby. It's okay to be a little chubby.

I have ZERO cosmetic products. I do not use deodorant. I do not use sunscreen. I do not use laundry detergent.

Guess who is aging better. I look about 15 years younger than her. When we got married, she was a superfox, 10/10; now she puts her hopes in wrinkle creams that don't work.

I told her to become a vegan, and she is trying to move in that direction, but she doesn't read books.

I think a person has to read books.

When you read about nutrition, and estrogen, and cancer, it's obvious that the best strategy is to become a low fat, vegan, cosmetic minimalist.

Advanced discussion of Cancer

Monoclonal origin

- Cancer is thought to arise from a single cell of origin.
- Human cells normally work together for the benefit of the entire body.
- Cancer cells have broken out of the normal, altruistic mode, and now are just reproducing in their own "selfish" mode.
- Cell growth = cell gets bigger.
- Cell division = cell replicates.

Contact inhibition = normal cells express cell surface chemicals, that tell other cells adjacent to them, that they should not replicate; to prevent crowding.

- Cancer is human cells behaving badly; like bacteria; out for themselves, instead of for the whole organism.

- **Presumed carcinogens** = tobacco, alcohol, estrogenic chemicals, aluminum, benzene, aflatoxin, tumor viruses (HBV, HCV), oils, meat.

Cancer causation by mutation is called the **"Somatic Mutation Theory" or SMT.**

- SMT says that somatic cells (means non-germ cells) undergo mutations;
    - the mutations enable them to proliferate out of control.
- Most cancers are thought to originally come from one cell; and this is called the "monoclonal origin of a tumor."
    - However, mutations occur within the cells of a malignant tumor.

- Cancers eventually tend to develop a **wide variety of mutations.**
    - The same tumor can have different mutations in different cells, and this is called **"intra-tumoral heterogeneity."**

    - Intra-tumoral heterogeneity can decrease the likelihood of response to monotherapy.

    - Tumoral heterogeneity is a major problem.

    - Tumoral heterogeneity means that CANCER tends to become MORE AGGRESSIVE over time.

    - The bigger the tumor gets, the more mutated it tends to get.

    - Cancer can turn into an uncontrollable monster.

The point is that you want to prevent it if possible, and certainly **do NOT give it any tumor promoters.**

- No meat. Not one bite.
- That means no milk, no cheese, no yogurt, no fish. Not one bite.
- No oils. That includes no olive oil. Not one drop.

- No alcohol. Not one sip.
- No tobacco. Not one puff.
- I've seen tons of people die from cancer.
- The best option is to try to prevent it.
- If you already have it, then optimize your health to perfection, and hopefully you will be able to slow it down.
- Lots of studies show that optimizing health by optimizing nutrition (most important thing), exercise, sunshine, social support, purpose, and avoiding psychological stress, can often lead to a big improvement in outcome.

The rationale goes like this:

Okay, Mr Cancer, you may have made a little spot for yourself inside of me, but I'm gonna make you wish you were somewhere else.

- I will NOT give you any tumor promoters.

- I will alkalinize your milieu with plant foods.

- I will increase oxygen delivery by eating a low fat, low salt plant food diet.

- I will also increase oxygen delivery with exercise.

- I will improve immune function with exercise.

- I will lower cortisol by avoiding unnecessary stress and caffeine.

- I will be nice to people, and maintain my social support, so that I can spend more time in a parasympathetic mood, which improves healing.

- I will avoid milk and other excesses of calcium, and go out in the sun, to get more 1,25-hydroxy vitamin D — the active form.

- I will help at least one other person every day, for their sake, and for

150

mine, because somehow being good to others, energizes our souls to want to live.

"Believe that life is worth living, and your belief will help create the fact."
                                                                    - William James.

"Does faith spring from miracles, or do miracles spring from faith?"
                                                                    - Dostoevsky.

My Mom had a 2 year prognosis, but lived 11 years.

She did great with all the social stuff; minister of care, director of an orphanage, tour guide for art museum, tour guide for architecture, tennis player, charming, funny personality.

But she screwed up by continuing to eat meat and oils. At the time, I didn't know enough to advise her.

- Critics of the SMT say that mitochondrial dysfunction — a metabolic problem — is the initiating event — that leads to mutations.
    - In other words, mitochondrial dysfunction leads to increased reactive oxygen species (ROS), and advanced glycation endproducts (AGEs);
    - and the ROS and AGE's then cause the mutations;
    - and that's why the mutation pattern is so variable.

- The Cancer Genome Atlas project (TCGA) showed that cancer mutations are relatively random.

Metabolic theory of cancer (MTC) posits that cancer is mostly driven by metabolic factors.

- Travis Christofferson wrote a book called "**Tripping over the truth**" about metabolic theory.
- Christofferson's book is a great book for pathophysiology — one of the best — but it screws up on diet recommendations.
- I actually do think it's a great book, and that all cancer patients should read it.
- Christofferson's book provides the scientific background to

understand cancer in a sophisticated way.

- Christofferson is really good at explaining the historical development of research into cancer related physiology, and genetics, and therapy.
- I was impressed by the entire book except the high fat diet recommendation.
- However, because of the importance of the topic, and the desire to help the cancer patients, I must correct the dietary recommendations of Seyfried and Christofferson.

Waarburg, Pederson, Hee Ko, Seyfried, McDougall and Campbell are some of the most famous researchers to promote the metabolic theory of cancer.

Otto Waarburg, biochemist noticed that different types of cancer all tended to produce lactic acid **(Waarburg effect).**

- Otto believed that cancer was primarily a **metabolic disease;**
- Otto believed that **hypoxia** causes **mitochondrial dysfunction.**
- Others, who agree with Waarburg, believe that mitochondrial dysfunction then leads to DNA **mutations**.
- Tissue hypoxia as could be caused by rouleaux of RBC's can lead to mitochondrial dysfunction.
- Saturated fat related excess intramyocellular lipid can lead to excess beta oxidation and excess NADH and FADH2 electron carriers going to electron transport.
- The excess electrons can lead to an excess voltage gradient across the inner mitochondrial membrane.
- The excess voltage gradient can lead to electon transport dysfunction which means mitochondrial dysfunction.
- Damaged mitochondria can die.
- Cancer cells have a diminished number of mitochondria.
- The remaining mitochondria are often abnormally small, or deformed in shape.

Cells with depleted mitochondria often die by necrosis or apoptosis.

The cancer cell is the rare cell that was hypoxic, but instead of dying by apoptosis, it mutated, and shifted

to anaerobic metabolism.

- In the process of becoming anaerobic, it **dedifferentiated**.
- To dedifferentiate means to stop caring about the cells around itself; to stop trying to be part of an organ like the breast, or the prostate, or the colon; **to only care about itself**;
- to only care about surviving itself, and to hell with it's old duties.
- The cancer cell has **REVERSE EVOLVED** to become like an anaerobic bacteria that just wants to grow as fast as it can,
- In order to grow it wants methionine, and leucine.

Cancer cells often induce or acquire certain metabolic patterns.

- **The mutation to increase hexokinase 2, also prevents apoptosis.**

Cancer types

- Cancer of an epithelial cell is called a **carcinoma**.
  - Most cancers are carcinomas, about 80%.
  - Epithelial cells are thought vulnerable to cancer, because they tend to have intrinsically high rates of cell replication.
- Cancer of lymphocytes is called a **lymphoma**.
- Cancer of connective tissues are called **sarcomas**, and are rare.
- Cancers of blood cells include **leukemias** and **myelomas**.
- Cancers of pigment cells are called **melanomas**.

*"The human body has an amazing capacity **to repair damaged DNA**. If this ability is supported through proper nutrition, most if not all of the damage can be undone long before cancer is initiated...*

Probably 97 to 98% of all cancers are related to diet and lifestyle, and not to genes...

None of the accepted "causes" of cancer in the absence of high animal protein diet mattered that much. Not genetics, not chemical carcinogens, not viruses." - TC Campbell from "Whole, rethinking science of nutrition."

Cancer Metabolism

- Accumulation of **lactic acid** suggests the cancer cells are generating energy from glycolysis in cytoplasm, rather than oxidative phosphorylation in mitochondria.

- **Anaerobic metabolism** enables a cancer cell to grow farther from capillaries;
    - Allows cancer cells to pump lactate into the extracellular space
    - causing acidosis
    - that can get adjacent cells to induce **ANGIOGENESIS**.

- Lactate accumulation can cause increased hypoxia inducible factor (HIF), which leads to increased VEGF for angiogenesis.

- Glycolysis provides substrates for cell replication.

- Anaerobic metabolism enables cell to survive even with mitochondrial dysfunction.

- Lactate can be sent to liver for conversion into glucose via gluconeogenesis.

- **One way to prevent angiogenesis is to PREVENT HYPOXIA.**

- **To prevent hypoxia you need to improve blood flow!!!**

- **To improve blood flow, you need to eat low fat, low salt, whole food, plant based diet.**

- *"**High fat meal decreases PO2 by 20%**... Waarburg said that he could turn normal cells in tissue culture into cancer cells by depriving them of oxygen."*   - John McDougall MD.

- **Some say glycolysis excess in cancer cells is mainly because the cell wants to use glycolytic intermediates for synthesis;**

- because dividing cells need more synthesis to get ready for cell duplication.

- **This is the main theory mentioned in current pathology textbooks.**

- Others say that the reason the cell relies on glycolysis, is because there is mitochondrial dysfunction.

  - Proponents of this theory believe, that if mitochondrial function could be improved,

  - then the patient would likely improve.

- F-DG PET scan is based on the Waarburg effect.
  - Cancer cells can take up 100x as much glucose as normal cells. This can lead to cachexia.
  - Waarburg effect helps cancer cells to grow in hypoxic conditions.

On the one hand, I admire Seyfried and Christofferson for improving knowledge of the metabolic theory of cancer.

On the other hand, I think they are wrong about recommending a high fat diet, because both saturated fat, and PUFA's are harmful to mitochondria.

Both saturated fat and PUFA's cause atherosclerosis, and atherosclerosis leads to hypoxia, and hypoxia favors cancer.

High fat diet means high meat diet, and high meat means high leucine, and methionine. Leucine and methionine appear to promote cancer growth.

High meat diet means increased metabolic acidosis, and acidosis favors cancer.

Seyfried and Christofferson have more direct experience in cancer research than I do, and can say that I'm just a blowhard who does not do research, and does not take care of cancer patients.

Even though that's true, I know I'm right.

Go ahead.

Read about it yourself.

- The **metabolic theory of cancer and the vegan diet** are not very popular because nobody makes money off them, and because most people are too ignorant to ever try to understand them.

- It would be easier to teach my dog sign language, than to get the average American to eat a vegan diet.

Metastasis

- **Metastases** = distant spread of cancer.
- Metastasis is the main reason that people die from cancer.
- Cancer kills by metastasis.

Metastasis is a multistep process that includes:

- Enlargement of the tumor size, beyond 2 mm, requires angiogenesis.
- Hypoxia of a tumor leads to increased HIF (Hypoxia Inducible Factor). Vitamin C helps prevent HIF activation.
- Increased HIF leads to increased VEGF (Vascular Endothelial Growth Factor).
- Metastatic spread requires that the tumor detaches from adjacent tumor cells.
- The cancer cell must then invade its own epithelial basement membrane.
- The cancer cell must then lyse its way through the adjacent extracellular matrix (ECM) connective tissue.
- Vitamin C helps make strong collagen, which might make it harder for cancer cells to lyse their way through ECM.

- Once the cancer cell has travelled through the ECM, it has to dig its way through the endothelial, basement membrane, tight junctions.

- Then the cancer cell has to INTRAvasate itself into a vein or lymphatic vessel.

- The cancer cell interacts with the immune system in the blood, and the lymphatics, and must survive this.

- The cancer cell is carried to its metastatic destination which is most often the lung, but can be anywhere including the liver, bones, or brain.

- Tumor must now repeat the above process in reverse = EXTRAVAsate into ECM.

    - Travel through ECM.
    - Grow in new location.
    - Induce angiogenesis.

- These are a lot of steps. That's why it usually takes decades for cancer to grow and metastasize.

- That's why a person should try to "slow down" the cancer by optimizing their health.

- **<u>Standard treatments for cancer</u>**

    - Surgery for focal tumors.
    - Radiation for nonresectable tumors.
    - Chemotherapy for treatment of primary tumors, micrometastases, and macrometastases.

<u>Cancer cell properties:</u>

- Mutations are common like in P53 gene.

- Cell might have problem with DNA repair. Vitamin C helps maintain DNA.

- **Cell might be overstimulated by growth factors like:**

    - ILGF 1 = increased by animal protein.
    - Insulin = increased by fat = meat and oils.
    - Estrogen = increased by meat.
    - Estrogenic chemicals = EDC's

- Mitochondrial dysfunction.
- Dependence on amino acids like those more common in meat.
- Grows in a hypoxic, acidotic milieu.

Why is the milieu acidic?

- Because cancer cells primarily produce energy from glycolysis.
- Glycolysis generates NADH. But the NADH has "nowhere to go." The NADH cannot send its electrons to electron transport, because mitochondria are dysfunctional.
- Therefore, the cell needs to find a new way to regenerate NAD+, so it can keep running glycolysis.
- Glycolysis requires NAD+ to run.
- The cancer cell solves the problem by converting pyruvate to **lactate**.
- During the conversion of pyruvate to lactate, NAD+ is regenerated.
- The lactate is then secreted into the extracellular matrix to create an acidotic milieu.
- The acidotic milieu favors growth of the cancer cell relative to other cells.
- The acidotic milieu also deactivates immune system cells — CD8 T cells and NK cells — which protects the cancer cells from the immune system.
- To some extent, cancer can be thought of as **reverse embryology** and **reverse evolution**.
- Cancer cells are "immortal" and can keep dividing; cancer cells have telomerase, and do not have a **Hayflick limit**.
- Cancer cells have uncontrolled proliferation, behaving like bacteria.
- Normal cells exposed to hypoxia have a tendency to die by necrosis or apoptosis.
- Cancer cells are unique in their overproduction of **hexokinase 2**;

  - Hexokinase 2 binds to mitochondria.
  - Hexokinase 2 blocks mitochondrial induced apoptosis.
  - Hexokinase 2 sucks up glucose like a vacuum cleaner.
  - Cancer cells burn through tons of glucose, and that's why cancer cells are hot on FDG PET.
  - Remember, that the glucose levels in diabetes are high because the fat has messed up glucose metabolism, NOT

158

because the patient eats glucose.

- Cancer cells have a massive uptake of glucose. Cancer cells use glucose for energy, and for synthesis.

- When glucose enters the cell, it is phosphorylated to become glucose 6-phosphate. Glucose 6-phosphate is of course the beginning of glycolysis.

- Glucose 6-phosphate can be diverted into the **pentose phosphate pathway (PPP)**.

- **PPP is also called Hexose MonoPhosphate (HMP) shunt.**

- PPP is used to make ribose for DNA and RNA synthesis.

- To replicate itself, a cell must make a copy of it's DNA; all **3.2 billion base pairs**. That's a lot of **ribose**.

    - That requires a lot of nitrogen for nucleotide bases, the purines and pyrimidines.
    - That requires a lot of PROTEIN intake.
    - That requires a lot of methionine, and leucine.

Phospholipid synthesis

- For replication, cancer cells also have to make a lot of phospholipids for **plasma cell membranes**, and membranes of organelles.
- Glycolysis provides dihyroxyacetone phosphate (**DHAP**) to serve as the carbon skeleton backbone for phospholipids.

- Cell has to replicate its contents:

    - Protein 55%
    - Nucleic acids 25%
    - Lipids 15%
    - CHO 5%

HYPOXIA

159

- Rouleaux causes mild hypoxia.

- Rouleaux reduces PO2 by 20%.

- Most people have a large amount of reserve, so a 20% drop in PO2 is not noticed by them.

- But, in elderly patients with comorbidities, 20% drop in PO2 is a big deal.

- Hypoxia causes upregulation of **Hypoxia Inducible Factor (HIF).**

    - HIF is a transcription factor.

- **HIF-1** activates genes for **INCREASED SYNTHESIS OF GLUT 1 & 3 TRANSPORTERS** to increase the basal rate of glucose uptake by cancer cells.

- Increased glut 1 & 3 transporters enables the cancer cell to survive better than "normal cells," in a hypoxic milieu.

- HIF-1 activates production of **INCREASED ENZYMES FOR GLYCOLYSIS**, including hexokinase, phosphofructokinase (PFK), and aldolase.

    - This increases glycolysis in the cell.
    - Cancer runs on **glycolysis**.

- HIF also increases production of **Pyruvate DeHydrogenase Kinase (PDHK-1).**

- PDHK-1 inhibits Pyruvate DeHydrogenase (PDH).

    - Thus, pdhK blocks the conversion of pyruvate by PDH into acetyl Coa.
    - Thus PDHK-1 **blocks the forward direction of the TCA (TriCarboxylic Acid) cycle (also known as Kreb's cycle).**
    - Thus pdhK pushes the cell to run on GLYCOLYSIS.

- **HIF causes increased glycolysis, and decreased Kreb's cycle** (in the forward direction).

- **Thus hypoxia can push the cell to running on glycolysis like a cancer cell!**

- HIF also induces increased secretion of **VEGF (Vascular Endothelial Growth Factor)** leading to **angiogenesis** — production of new blood vessels — that enables cancer cells to keep growing — and enables the cancer cells to metastasize!

- Prevent angiogenesis, and you prevent metastasis.

- Prevent hypoxia, and you might prevent angiogenesis.

- **Mutations** sometimes occur in the **enzymes** of **Kreb's cycle** called succinate dehydrogenase and fumarase making them less functional; which leads to accumulation of proximal, Kreb's cycle substrates like succinate and fumarate; which turn out to be inhibitors of **prolyl hydroxylase 2**.

- Normally, prolyl hydroxylase 2 functions to degrade HIF. When prolyl hydroxylase is inhibited by succinate and fumarate, that means that HIF 1 stays active.

- **Lactate accumulation** also inhibits prolyl hydroxylase 2, and thus prolongs the activation of HIF.

- Thus hypoxia alone can shift a cell into glycolysis based metabolism, and angiogenesis.

- Mutations in **Isocitrate DeHydrogenase** (IDH) lead to production of **2-hydroxy glutarate**.

- Normal enzyme isocitrate dehydrogenase converts isocitrate into alpha ketoglutarate.

- 2 hydroxy glutarate is considered an "onco-metabolite." 2 hydroxy glutarate **changes DNA methylation**, leading to the cell becoming **less dependent on growth factors**; in other words, the cell is

dedifferentiating; going backwards in embryologic time;

- backwards in evolutionary time; instead of being a functional part of an organ, that is a functional part of a human, the cell is now on its own;

- just trying to grow independent of the adjacent cells.

- Insulin, insulin like growth factor, and estrogen are all growth factors.

- Normal cells only grow when get a signal from a growth factor that they should grow.

- **IDH mutation gets cells to grow even with relative lack of growth factors apparently**.

- There is evidence that if cancer cells can have electron transport & oxidative phosphorylation restored, the cancer cell might stop behaving like cancer, and restart to behave like a normal cell.

- Vitamin C helps to degrade HIF.
    - Vitamin C is an antioxidant that comes from plants.

OBESITY

- Fat people have increased sleep apnea which can lead to tissue hypoxia.
- Fatness is usually due to eating meat (animal protein + saturated fat), vegetable oils, and exposures to EDC's.

- **NIGHT SHIFT WORK.**

    - Body perceives lack of sleep as stress.
    - Chronic, excess psychological stress leads to chronic high cortisol.
- Chronic high cortisol can damage neurons in the hippocampus, and lead to cognitive decline.
- Messes up circadian rhythm.

Chapter 12

Iron, ferroptosis,and neurodegeneration

What is the key point about iron?

In medical school, everyone learns about iron deficiency anemia.

It's a ho-hum, snoozer topic.

In women, it's usually from abnormal uterine bleeding.

In men, it's often from colon cancer.

The big insight is that a lot more people suffer from **IRON OVERLOAD**, than iron deficiency; and hardly anyone knows this.

Why is iron overload important?

In the movies, death is often a dramatic event, due to the fatal flaw of the tragic hero.

In real life, people usually get nickeled and dimed to death. Unhealthy forces vandalize their body parts; chipping away, destroying their cognitive function, immune system, and physical strength.

Then they fall, and break a hip, or bleed into their brains, or catch a cold, and have an accelerated decline to death.

What is meant by "nickeled and dimed?"

Sickness is easy to understand when $2 + 2 = 4$. Everyone gets this.

Sickness is challenging to understand when $1.3 + 2.2 + .8 + 4.7 = 9$; but that is the more common pattern of sickness.

To understand a disease, one should study each of the causes.

Why study the causes of disease?

Because, once you understand them, you are better able to avoid them.

The best way to prevent a disease, is to avoid the things that cause it.

What is ferroptosis?

Ferro means iron. Ptosis means falling off. Ferroptosis means cell death due to iron.

Why am I scared of ferroptosis?

Let's say you get ferroptosis in your bone marrow derived, endothelial cell precursors (EPC's); those are your endothelial "stem cells."

If you destroy your EPC's, then your risk of atherosclerosis just went way up!!!

A smart person tries to maintain their physiologic reserve.

How does iron cause ferroptosis?

Iron is a transitional metal, which means it has a variable valence, typically Fe^{2+} (ferrOUS) or Fe^{3+} (ferrIC).

Ferr"OUS" reminds me of "deuce" for 2.

Ferr"IC" with the "i" pronounced like the long vowel sound for "e" reminds me of thr"EE" which also has a long vowel sound for "e."

Variable valence enables iron to help enzymes catalyze chemical reactions.

Normally the body tries to keep iron bound to proteins.

Iron is transported in the blood bound to transferrin.

Iron is stored in cells bound to ferritin.

Iron does a great service to us in hemoglobin, cytochromes, and other enzymes.

164

When is iron a problem?

Iron is a problem when it's breaks loose from proteins; iron on it's own is called free iron, or labile iron, or unliganded iron.

Why is free iron a problem?

Because free iron can become autocatalytic with Fenton, and Haber Weiss chemistry.

In the Fenton reaction, Fe catalyzes conversion of H_2O_2 into $O_2^{\bullet-}$ (superoxide anion).

Autocatalytic iron can generate lots of reactive oxygen species (ROS).

What is the significance of iron related ROS?

Intracellular iron related ROS can lead to ferroptosis.

Brent Stockwell PhD is one of the best experts on ferroptosis.

Extracellular iron related ROS can lead to distortion of RBC's, and fibrinogen, leading to hypercoaguability, and neurodegeneration.

The free iron can be taken up by dormant bacteria in our blood, and these may release LPS.

Do we have dormant bacteria in our blood?

Yes, we do have some bacteria that are dormant in our blood.

Bacterial dormancy shouldn't be that surprising. We know that TB, syphilis, and Lyme disease can be dormant.

We know that some bacteria can form dormant endospores.

We know that viruses like herpes can be dormant, and be reactivated by psychological stress.

We know that the catecholamine stress hormones can function as siderophores to permit increased bacterial uptake of iron.

When free iron is available, some of these bacteria can come out of dormancy.

Douglas Kell PhD is one of the best experts on iron related neurodegeneration, and how it relates to stroke, and Alzheimer's disease.

Kell wrote a great paper called, "Iron behaving badly."

What happens during ferroptosis?

Free iron generates ROS.

The ROS react with PUFA's (Poly Unsaturated Fatty Acids) to cause a chain reaction of lipid peroxidation.

Lipid peroxidation involving the plasma membrane can cause cell death.

Lipid peroxidation of the mitochondrial membrane can cause mitochondrial dysfunction, and lead to cell death.

What are some common PUFA's in humans?

- Linoleic acid.
- Arachidonic acid.
- Cardiolipin.
- EPA.
- DHA.

Why PUFA's?

PUFA's are much more susceptible to lipid peroxidation, than are saturated fats. PUFA's are more susceptible, because the methylene bridge carbon is only weakly bound to carbon.

What is a methylene bridge carbon?

The typical omega 6 fatty acid has double bonds on carbon #6, and carbon #9.

C1—C2—C3—C4—C5—C6==C7—**C8**—C9==C10—C11—C12—C13 —C14—C15—C16==O, —OH.

Carbon #8, C8, is the methylene bridge carbon. C8 has only a WEAK bond to hydrogen. ROS can react with C8 to initiate lipid peroxidation.

The C8 lipid peroxide can then start a chain reaction that destroys other fatty acids. These fatty acids can be part of plasma membranes or mitochondrial membranes.

When the plasma membrane is disrupted, the cell cannot maintain its gradients distinct from the extracellular space, and the cell dies.

When the mitochondrial membrane(s) are disrupted, the mitochondria cannot maintain its intramembranous space proton gradient, and they can't make energy with ATP synthase.

When mitochondria can't make energy, the cell usually dies.

Ferroptosis is cell death, due to free iron related ROS, leading to lipid peroxidation.

The methylene bridge carbon is also sometimes called the "bis-allylic" carbon. Bis means two (for the two double bonds near it). "Allyl" comes from the fact that "garlic" has a chemical structure like this.

Why do people store so much iron?

I think it's because our ancestors were at risk for bleeding due to trauma. Storage iron enabled them to quickly resynthesize hemoglobin.

Why do people become overloaded?

Children are unlikely to become iron overloaded, because they are growing fast.

Women of reproductive age are unlikely to become iron overloaded, because of menstruation.

Adult men and postmenopausal women are at increased risk for iron overload, because they have no good way to get rid of iron.

They lose a little iron by sloughing off some skin.

Where does iron come from?

Meat iron is bound to hemoglobin. A large percentage of dietary meat iron — heme iron — is absorbed from the gut into the blood.

Heme iron absorption is related to dietary meat intake; eat more meat, and you will absorb more iron.

Plants do not have hemoglobin. The gut is much better at regulating absorption of plant iron. Only a relatively small percentage of plant iron is absorbed from the gut into the blood.

Thus, meat eaters tend to become iron overloaded. It takes decades for this to occur.

How else does iron become free?

Iron becomes free when cells die from necrosis. During necrosis, cell contents leak out, including ferritin.

Ferritin is normally located inside of cells. Ferritin is a giant molecule that stores over 4,000 molecules of iron.

Liver cells store a lot of ferritin. Necrosis of a liver cell can "spill" a lot of iron into the blood.

What can prevent ferroptosis?

Avoid eating **vegetable oils** —which are really seed oils — because these contain lots of **PUFA's**.

Avoid **meat** to decrease **iron** load on the body. Avoiding meat also lowers saturated fat intake, which makes life easier for mitochondria, so they will have more reserve, to be able to fend off iron related ROS.

What about the dangers of fructose from processed foods?

Avoid sweetened beverages, because of the excess fructose. Fructose from processed foods goes to the liver, and gets converted into fat.

This fat then causes insulin resistance with reversal of electron transport. The reversal of electron transport, leads to a blockage of glycolysis, which leads to accumulation of methyl glyoxal (MGO).

MGO forms AGE's (Advanced Glycation Endproducts) which bind R-AGE (Receptor for AGE's). R-AGE activates NADPH oxidase which causes increased ROS, and oxidative stress.

Excess fructose also causes problems via uric acid (urate). When the junk food bolus of fructose enters liver cells, it gets converted to Fructose 1-Phosphate. The phosphate comes from ATP which ends up as AMP. The AMP gets converted to Inosine MonoPhosphate (IMP), and then to hypoxanthine, xanthine, and finally to uric acid.

This excess of uric acid leads to decreased endothelial Nitric Oxide Synthase (eNOS), and therefore decreased nitric oxide. Decreased endothelial nitric oxide is associated with vasoconstriction, and hypertension (HTN).

Uric acid also leads to increased activation of NADPH oxidase, and resultant increase in ROS, and oxidative stress.

Uric acid is also thought to be prothrombotic via probably acting as a "bridging molecule" between RBC's to cause rouleaux formation, according to Dr Gregory Sloop, the great atherosclerosis researcher.

What about the benefits of fruits?

Increase consumption of fruits to increase vitamin C levels. Vitamin C is an antioxidant that helps to quench ROS.

Plants have lots of **antioxidants** that help you to quench ROS. Meat has almost no antioxidants, because the animal has already used them up.

Plants need to make antioxidants, so they can survive being out in the sun all day.

If it's too hot and sunny outside, then animals can just WALK into the shade. Animals also have fur to block the sun.

The color of fruits and vegetables indicates their antioxidants. Orange in carrots and sweet potatos indicates beta carotene. Red in tomatos indicates lycopene.

Green leafy vegetables have lots of antioxidants.

Probably the main reason we have color vision is for eating fruits, and being able to see when they're ripe.

You can donate blood — therapeutic phlebotomy — to decrease your iron load.

In the future, iron chelation may play a role in preventing ferroptosis.

How much blood should a person donate?

I don't know. I have not yet donated blood, but I'm thinking about it.

The older you get, the more fragile you get.

Up til now, I'm still pretty healthy with a fasting, total cholesterol of 105-120. My energy is good. Yesterday I squatted 100 lbs for 100 reps. (Yes, that was 100 reps). PR interval is okay with the old lady.

Whenever I feel like I'm declining in a health variable, then I make an effort to add a new health habit.

So far, my strategy has been to just avoid eating meat, but if I sense a drop in my energy level, then my next step would be to check blood level of ferritin.

"Normal" ranges for ferritin have a wide range along the lines of 12-350. It's probably better to aim for a ferritin between 15-75.

Ferritin is normally supposed to be inside cells, and not in the blood. So blood level of ferritin is an indicator of cell necrosis.

The higher the ferritin level, the higher the risk of iron related autocatalytic activity, generation of ROS, and oxidative stress.

What about glutathione?

Glutathione is part of the antioxidant system. Glutathione is a tripeptide of glutamate-glycine-cysteine (G-G-C).

What are some of the most important antioxidants?

Vitamin C, vitamin E, glutathione, glutathione peroxidase, coenzyme Q10.

What do antioxidants do?

- Antioxidants work together as a network of reducing power.
- Antioxidants donate electrons to quench free radicals.
- Free radicals want electrons. Free radicals steal electrons.
- Antioxidants are able to donate an electron, and then remain stable themselves.
- Pathogens are usually oxidants; they oxidize other molecules, by stealing electrons from them.
- Antioxidants are anti-oxidation. Antioxidants are reducing agents.
- The more antioxidants a cell has, the more "reducing" power it has. When a molecule receives an electron, it's valence number decreases; it is REDUCED.
- If the antioxidants in a cell are depleted, then the cell is not be able to handle ROS.
- Therefore, adequate intake of fruits helps a cell to maintain its vitamin C level. Vitamin C can directly quench free radicals. Vitamin C can also reactivate vitamin E.
- Once an antioxidant has donated an electron, it needs to be reactivated itself; this is a form of "recycling."

How are free radicals drawn?

171

- Molecular oxygen is O_2
- Superoxide anion is $O_2 \cdot^-$
- H_2O_2 is not a free radical, but it can be converted into a free radical.
  - H_2O_2 made in the mitochondria, is able to exit the mitochondria;
  - this can lead to side effects distant from the mitochondria, like DNA mutations.
  - Guanine is especially vulnerable to ROS induced mutation, with the formation of 8-oxo-guanine.
- Hydroxyl radical is $HO \cdot$ → hydroxyl radical is superreactive, so tends to react locally.
- Peroxyl radical is $ROO \cdot$
- Lipid peroxide is R-OO-H

How does this relate to neurodegeneration?

Neuronal cell membranes have a significant amount of desirable PUFA's in the form of omega 3, EPA and DHA, which makes them vulnerable to lipid peroxidation.

Iron overload can also lead to hypercoaguability, which can plug up arteries in the brain.

Normally, the human body tries to keep iron liganded — sequestered — so that it is NOT available to bacteria.

Bacteria need iron to grow. Iron sequestration is a useful strategy for prevention of bacterial infections.

Iron overload can also make iron available to dormant bacteria in the blood. Once reawakened, these dormant bacteria can release some LPS, and this worsens hypercoaguability.

This combination of iron overload induced ROS, and hypercoaguabliity, and dormant bacteria reactivation seems to play a role in the making beta amyloid plaques become insoluble; thus accelerating development of Alzheimer's.

172

Chapter 13

Obesity

In the Victorian age, women wore dresses that made their butts stick out like car trunks. Nowadays, a lot of women really have butts that big.

What's the number one advice for fat people?

Get off your lazy asses, and read a book!

Why do you say that?

Because obesity is easy to cure if a person knows what they are doing.

Low fat, plant eaters are skinny.

Meat eaters are fat, usually.

I know the psychology of fat people, because I was one.

"Trust one who has been through it."   - Virgil.

What is the psychology of fat people?

At first, they try to lose the weight.

They try to exercise more, and eat less; but that NEVER works.

"Exercise more and eat less" is the mantra of chumps.

I tried that for four years and failed, and I've got as much willpower and brains as anyone on planet earth.

Then people start saying to themselves, "Oh well, I guess it's genetic. Maybe, I should just accept it as fate, that I'm supposed to be a fat person."

Then they see an article about a fad diet. They try it, and initially make progress for a month or two, then slip back into fatness, and despair.

This goes on for a couple of years. Their families make fun of them. Their peers make fun of them. Strangers make fun of them.

What are they supposed to do?

Read about epidemiology.

Why epidemiology?

They will discover that rice eaters are always skinny.

They will learn that the average bmi of a low fat vegan is around 22.

They will learn the Tarahumara are skinny. The Okinawans are skinny. The vegan 7th day adventists are skinny. The Yanomamo are skinny. The Tsimane are skinny.

Low salt populations — like Yanomamo of South America, Xingu of Brazil, Papua New Guinea, Australian Aborigines, and rural Kenyans — have very low risk of hypertension.

Plant foods are low in sodium, and high in potassium. Potassium is a vasodilator, which helps to lower blood pressure.

The Tsimane of Bolivia, who eat their original, endemic diets are much healthier, with much less atherosclerosis. Some Tsimane were encouraged to get calcium heart CT scans, and they had the lowest coronary calcium scores, ever recorded.

You don't need will power. You don't need to exercise. You don't need a fad diet.

You just need to eat a low fat, vegan diet.

What does "low fat" vegan mean?

Vegan means only eat plants; 100% plants. Zero% animal foods.

Low fat means:

No oils.
No nuts.
No seeds.

Oils are not food. Oils are a poison. Even olive oil is bad for you.

Olive oil is not just monounsaturated fat. Olive oil also often contains over 10% saturated fat. Even if it were just monounsaturated fat, it would still be bad for you.

Oil means liquid fat. Oil means high caloric density with no fiber. Eating fat makes you fat.

The human body is NOT made to eat liquid fat.

Oils screw up metabolism, and make you sick; oils typically contain omega 6 PUFA's (Poly Unsaturated Fatty Acids) that predispose you to lipid peroxidation, and they increase inflammation via excess arachidonic acid.

The most common omega 6 fatty acid you will hear about is linoleic acid, C18:2, 6, 9. The numbers indicate double bonds beginning on carbons 6 and 9, counting from the methyl end of the fatty acid.

Omega 6 fatty acids are tumor promoters.

Corn has omega 6 fats. Feed lot animals — who are fed corn — will have relatively high levels of omega 6 fats.

Even the omega 3 oils appear to be associated with increase risk of prostate cancer, and potentially other types of increased cancer risk.

Excess intake of omega 3 supplements might suppress the immune system, and make it less able to prevent cancer.

Better to just eat plants, and let your gut decide how much omega 3's to absorb. Plants have ALA (Alpha Linolenic Acid), and your body can convert ALA to EPA, and DHA.

The most common omega three fatty acid you will hear about is alpha linolenic acid, C 18:3, 3, 6, 9. The numbers indicate double bonds beginning on carbons 3, 6 and 9, counting from the methyl end of the fatty acid.

Humans are not made to eat oils! Oils are an industrial produced toxin.

The purpose of nuts and seeds are for a plant to reproduce itself. Nuts and seeds are mostly fat. Fat is a concentrated source of calories.

Animal fat is worse than plant fat, but plant fat in large amounts is still bad for arteries. Most "nut eaters" don't eat just a "few" nuts; they eat large handfuls of nuts.

Caldwell Esselstyn MD — the doctor with the best results in the world for prevention of coronary artery disease — tells his patients, "No nuts."

Esselstyn of course also tells his patients, "No oil."

Nowadays, you will hear some younger doctors say, "A few nuts are okay. A little bit of Olive oil is okay."

My advice is to stick with what Esselstyn recommends — no nuts and no oil — he's got the best results in the world for preventing coronary artery disease. He's in his 80's, but still fit and smart. He's knows what he's doing.

What's the point?

If a person wants to be skinny, they should eat what skinny people eat.

Skinny people satisfy their hunger with starch or fruits.

That's it.

Be a starchivore, or a fruitarian, and you will be skinny.

The converse is also true.

Eat any other way, and you will stay fat.

Hold on a second. Haven't lots of people lost weight in other ways?

Yes, but that's usually only short term.
Short term results are irrelevant.

The goal is to be slim and healthy for the rest of your life.

Short term, a person can lose weight with any diet.

It's called the Hawthorne effect — which is also called the observer effect.

When a person is being observed, and their performance measured, they try harder. When a person is in a diet study, they pay closer attention to what they are eating.

When the newness wears off, they slip back into fatness.

Fad diets are difficult to maintain for more than 3 months.

What about the low fat vegan diet? Isn't the low fat vegan diet a fad?

No. The low fat vegan diet has been the most common way for humans to eat, since the beginning of humans.

The low fat vegan diet is easy to sustain for the rest of one's life.

Take a look at a fish. Just the fish. Do you really want to eat that?

It's disgusting. Would you eat a bit of a raw fish, just by itself.

I wouldn't.

To make a fish edible, it has to be cooked, and then salted, and spiced, and soaked in Ketchup or tartar sauce or something.

If you see a bowl of fruit on a table, you salivate. You don't need to modify it in any way.

We are made to eat fruit.

What about starch?

The agricultural expansion was about 10,000 years ago. And we had fire by that time.

Cooked starch became the most common way for people to eat. Since the beginning of recorded time, humans have eaten most of their calories in the form of cooked starch.

All the healthy populations get the majority of their calories from cooked starch.

What are examples of cooked starch?

Rice, potatos, sweet potatos, quinoa, squash, beans, peas, green beans, oatmeal, corn, pumpkin.

What is the best rice?

Organic is preferable.

Avoid rice from areas that used to grow cotton, because it often used to be sprayed with arsenic.

I still routinely eat rice, but only organic, from low arsenic areas.

I would never eat chicken, because besides being a meat, it has a much higher risk of high arsenic levels.

Take home message:

Most fat people don't know about the 100% plant based diet, and that's why they are fat.

Being fat after fifty is like walking around with a neon sign that says, "got HTN, DM, CAD, ED, cognitive impairment."

Attention: Fatso's of the world unite, and convert to veganism. You have nothing to lose, but your diabetes needles.

It's time for your vegan renaissance. You can become "born again" vegans.

Here's a conversation between a doctor, and an imaginary patient named Chumpy Dumas (as in Dum-azz).

Chumpy: What should I do now?

Doctor: You need to lose weight?

Chumpy: You don't think I've tried every g_dd_mn, f_cking diet!?#!^!

Do you think I want to be fat!?#!^!

Doctor: Calm down, Chumpy.

I understand.

Most people fail at dieting, because they don't know what they are doing.

Chumpy: Oh, c'mon Doc. Everybody knows you just

gotta exercise more, and eat less.

Doctor: Did that work for you?

Chumpy: No.

Doctor: It doesn't work for anybody.

You can't change the amount you eat. Your brain has a hypothalamic hunger center that is like a thermostat — with a **set point**.

The "thermostat" in your brain makes you eat — exactly the amount of your current foods — that you do.

You might try to overcome it with willpower, but that only works for a couple of days or weeks, months at the most.

Then a person starts binge-ing, and goes back to their baseline.

Chumpy: Okay. So, what should I do?

Doctor: You need to CHANGE what you eat.

When you CHANGE what you eat, you CHANGE the set point.

Chumpy: What should I eat?

Doctor: I've got one word for ya, Kid: PLANTS. Eat PLANTS.

When people eat a whole food, plant based diet with starches to satisfy their hunger, they are skinny.

How to optimize body weight:

Good foods to eat:

Become a 100% vegan.

100% vegan diet — whole foods, organic, starch and fruit based — is the healthiest diet in the world.

To optimize health, one should strive toward becoming 100% vegan.

Satisfy your hunger with starches like oatmeal, quinoa, potatos, sweet potatos, rice, beans, corn, squash, organic whole grains.

You can also satisfy your hunger with fruits.

Eat vegetables for nutrients.

Eat at least one salad per day, preferably two or three.

Avoid nuts because they are 70-90% fat.

Avoid seeds and avocados because they are high fat.

Bad foods = should always avoid:

Oils including olive oil and coconut oil. All oils are liquid fat.

Junk food = processed food with no fiber = usually has four or more bad ingredients = often contains oils, food dyes, MSG, excess salt, bad preservatives.

Meat. Meat includes milk, cheese, yogurt, ice cream.

Food additives that should be avoided:

<u>Salt</u>, because causes hypertension.

<u>MSG</u>, because appears to cause junk food addiction, and appears to sometimes cause headaches and insomnia.

Sodium benzoate, BHA, BHT.

Food dyes.

Food dyes are named with cute little euphemisms like Red #40.

Check out their chemical structures. Many of them are unhealthy petroleum based chemicals.

There are lots of articles on side effects of food dyes.

Don't eat anything with food dyes.

Do not feed junk food to your kids.

Once kids get into the habit of eating junk food, it's a lot harder to get them to eat healthy food.

Bad beverages:

Soda pop is all bad. Soda pop tends to contain:

Caffeine — to make you dehydrated and thirsty —

Salt — to make you hyperosmolar and thirsty —

Fructose — to cover up the taste of the salt.

Tea can concentrate fluoride and aluminum. I would never drink it. Tea is potentially neurotoxic. Tea also contains caffeine.

Caffeine can cause hypertension, which causes **atherosclerosis**.

Caffeine can cause **insomnia**. Lack of sleep leads to cravings for sweets which our ancestors probably tried to satisfy with fruits, but moderns tend to satisfy with sweets. Lack of sleep can cause **hyperglycemia**.

Caffeine is a trimethyl xanthine, and chemically related to purines. Caffeine can in some persons can exacerbate the effects of a folate or B12 deficiency.

Caffeine causes increased urinary excretion of **calcium**, which contributes to the risk of renal insufficiency, and kidney stones.

Caffeine causes increased urinary excretion of **magnesium**. Magnesium is your friend. Magnesium helps protect you from glutamate related neurotoxicity.

A lot of people are magnesium deficient. Plants are good sources of magnesium.

Caffeine is a mild, immunosuppressant. Caffeine mimics the acute stress response causing elevated adrenaline, noradrenaline, and cortisol. Cortisol is an immunosuppressant. Cortisol promotes obesity. It's difficult to lose weight when your sleep deprived, and cortisol levels are high.

Lack of sleep from insomnia causes increased cortisol. When cortisol levels are elevated, DHEA levels tend to be decreased.

The caffeine induced **catecholamines** can have a mild immunosuppressant effect by functioning as siderophores, to increase bacterial access to iron.

The human body prevents bacterial infection by sequestering iron.

Catecholamines are mildly prothrombotic.

What is the bottom line on caffeine?

In the short term, caffeine energizes you; that's good for obtaining your personal best with weight lifting; that's good if you're feeling sleepy, and you need to drive.

In the long term, caffeine is bad for you, because of the insomnia, hypertension, calciuria, magnesium loss in urine, and immunosuppression.

If you ask anyone, they will tell you, "I'd like to reduce my stress level."

Then they go and drink caffeine in the form of coffee, tea, or energy drink.

Brilliant! Caffeine closely mimics the **ACUTE STRESS RESPONSE**.

Similar to acute stress, caffeine increases cortisol, epinephrine (adrenaline),

183

blood pressure, heart rate, blood glucose, and blood total cholesterol. Then people will say, "Well, it's only for a little while."

But caffeine has a long half life —6-8 hours — and many persons drink 2 or more cups per day, so caffeine is active all day.

I recommend to completely avoid caffeine. If you feel that you must drink caffeine, then try to only drink caffeine for rare special occasions like trying to max out with weights, or being obligated to drive when you are sleepy.

I do not ever ingest any form of caffeine, including no coffee.

Chumpy: Coffee is bad?

Doctor: Yes.

Chumpy: Lots of healthy, smart people drink coffee.

Doctor: Yes, but they'd be healthier without it. Dr. Esselstyn has the best results of any doctor in the world, and he tells his patients to avoid caffeine.

Just look up the side effects of caffeine, and you won't want to drink it anymore.

I quit coffee years ago, and I felt better afterwards.

Chumpy: How can I lower my stress?

Doctor: Try to increase PANS (Parasympathetic Autonomic Nervous System), and decrease SANS (Sympathetic Autonomic Nervous System). Improve sleep. Body perceives lack of sleep as stress. Avoid caffeine. Avoid stressful people. Avoid stressful shows on TV. Avoid things that stress you out. Do things that you enjoy. Exercise. Try to spend time with positive people, and avoid negative people.

Parody of "Here we go round the mulberry bush."

Meat eater version:

- Bacon and eggs are for chumps,

- are for chumps, are for chumps.

- Bacon and eggs are for chumps.

  - on a cold and frosty morning.

- This is the way we fleece the proles,

  - fleece the proles, fleece the proles.

- This is the way we fleece the proles,

  - on a cold and frosty morning.

From the sermon by Veegus on Mount Broccoli

- *Two legs bad. Four legs bad. One stem good.*

- *Ye are the **starch** of the earth*

- *Ye shall know the truth, and the truth shall set ye free.*

- *Meat men are fat.*

- *Plant people are thin.*

Beatitudes

- **Blessed are they who are fat in belly,**

  - for they will be thin again.

- **Blessed are they who are poor in antioxidants,**

  - for they will improve a lot.

- **Blessed are they who have high blood viscosity,**

  - for they will get laminar flow.

- **Blessed are they who are hyper insulinemic,**

    - for they can improve response.

- **Blessed are they who want to learn,**

    - for they can be taught.

Why do people think nutrition is a joke?

And don't say it's because nutrition books have silly songs. They ate junk food from ages 5 to 35, and they looked okay. They don't realize that they've used up their reserve. Their aorta elastic fibers are gone. Their endothelial cell precursors – stem cells – are being depleted.

They are headed downhill fast if they don't change their ways.

Repent! Repent!

Most people are confused.

They hear contradictory information about food, and just figure, "No one really knows, so they might as well just eat whatever tastes good."

Big food wants it that way.

Most people don't know anyone who really knows nutrition.

"When I was a meat eater,

I spake as a meat eater,

I understood as a meat eater,

I thought as a meat eater:

but when I became a Vegan,

I put away **childish** things."   - First Corinthians 13:11.

186

Chapter 14

Leaky gut

What is leaky gut?

Leaky gut is when your gut has holes in it.

Holes in the gut lining allow absorption of big pieces of animal protein that can cause autoimmune disease.

Holes in the gut lining allow some bacterial endotoxins called LPS (Lipo Poly Saccharide) to pass through the gut wall and cause inflammation.

Why does the gut have holes in it? So what if big, pieces of protein are absorbed?

First we've gotta define some terms.

Meat is protein and fat.

Plants are carbohydrate and fiber.

- Normally, gastric acid prevents bacterial growth in the stomach and small bowel.

- Gut bacteria essentially means colon bacteria.

Why do we even have gut bacteria?

Good gut bacteria help us to digest our food.

Good gut bacteria help us to maintain our colon lining cells.

Good gut bacteria protect us from bad bacteria.

Good bacteria thrive on fiber.

The key to colon health is that plant fiber promotes good bacteria.

What is meant by "good" gut bacteria?

Fiber comes from plant foods. Good bacteria eat the fiber. Good bacteria make butyrate.

Colon enterocytes use the butyrate to make tight junctions, and prevent leaky gut.

What is meant by "bad" gut bacteria?

Bad diets – with meat and oils – lead to bad bacteria.

Bad bacteria worsen the gut lining, and increase the risk of inflammation, and autoimmune diseases. Bad bacteria are associated with increased LPS.

Bad bacteria deconjugate estrogen, leading to increased estrogen reabsorption, with increased risk of breast cancer, and prostate cancer.

Bad bacteria are associated with increased TMAO (TriMethyl Amine Oxide).   Bad bacteria are associated with increased colon cancer.

What is butyrate?

Butane is a four carbon alkane.

Butyric acid is a four carbon carboxylic acid.

Fatty acids are carboxylic acids.

Butyrate is the DEprotonated form of butyric acid.

In the medical literature, butyrate is often called a "short chain, fatty acid."

What is the most common nutrient deficiency?

Lack of fiber.

Lack of fiber associated with what diseases?

Abdominal pressure syndrome, gallstones, atherosclerosis, cancer, leaky gut.

In other words, almost all of the modern chronic diseases.

How much fiber should we eat?

Ideally, it is good to eat 100 grams of fiber per day or more.

What are the two main types of fiber?

Insoluble fiber is not soluble in water. Insoluble fiber is insoluble. Insoluble fiber just adds bulk to stool.

Soluble fiber is food for good gut bacteria.

Fiber comes from plants.

Meat has no fiber.

- Gut has two main types of bacteria.

    - **Bad bacteria** feed on meat.

    - **Good bacteria** feed on fiber from plants.

- When you eat plants; you get good bacteria; because good bacteria eat fiber.

- **Good bacteria** make the 4 carbon fatty acid called **butyrate**.

- Butyrate is the preferred food of the colon lining cells (enterocytes).

- Colon lining cells use the butyrate to make **TIGHT JUNCTIONS** between themselves.

- Thus, good bacteria help the colon lining cells — **enterocytes** — to maintain tight junctions between themselves.

- Tight junctions help maintain controlled absorption of proteins so you only absorb little pieces at a time.

- **Tight junctions** prevent big pieces of animal protein
    - from being absorbed.

- When you eat bad food = meat, oils, fried food, junk food, Frankenstein food; you get bad bacteria; because that's what they eat.

- Meat deprives the colon lining cells of butyrate, and the tight junctions are loosened.

- When a diet lacks fiber, the colon enterocyte inter-cellular junctions become **loose**.

- **Big chunks of animal protein** can be absorbed.

- Loose lips sink ships.

- Loose junction don't function.

- **Loose junctions** allow absorption of **animal protein chunks** that are **TOO BIG!**

- The body recognizes these as **foreign** invaders.

    - The body makes **antibodies** to the invading animal protein chunks.

- Animal proteins have similar amino acid sequences to human proteins; called **"molecular mimicry."**

- Therefore, the antibodies can "cross react" with similar sequences in the human body; called **"cross reactivity."**

- Leaky gut due to molecular mimicry,

- with antibody cross reactivity,

- is thought the main mechanism of **AUTOIMMUNE** disease.

- Autoimmune disease is a big deal. My best friend's mom died from Lupus.

- Autoimmune disease is common.

- Everybody knows someone with type one diabetes, or Hashimoto's thyroiditis, or Crohn's disease, or rheumatoid arthritis.

- Leaky gut might be the cause.

- Leaky gut tends to improve with vegan diet.

- 80% of autoimmune disease is in women overall.

- Meat has saturated fat and bacteria.
    - Saturated fat appears to facilitate passage of **bacterial endotoxin (LPS)** across our gut lining, and into our blood.

    - This is another mechanism of "leaky gut."

- Inflammatory diseases like gout,
    - and autoimmune diseases like Crohn's disease, rheumatoid arthritis and multiple sclerosis,
        - **are common in meat eaters**
        - **and rare in plant eaters.**

How long does it take to flip your colon from bad bacteria to good bacteria?

Just like the motto of the house renovation contractor: "Two weeks!"

When you switch from meats to beets, you get the farts for two weeks.

Leaky gut can also potentially contribute to psychiatric illness.

"All disease begins in the gut."   - Hippocrates.

*"The **invisible hand** of fiber protects your health."*   - Adam Smith.

The risk factors for leaky gut are:

- Meat.
- Vegetable oils.
  - Even whipped cream by itself causes leaky gut.

- Alcohol.
  - Alcohol is toxic to gut bacteria.
  - Alcohol is a tumor promoter.

- Antibiotics.
- Chlorinated water contributes. Can remove by carbon filter, or reverse osmosis filter.
- NSAIDs can cause leaky gut.

- Lack of fiber = lack of whole plant foods.
- Dishwasher soap that gets into your food.
  - Avoid by rinse dish before you eat off it.
  - Better yet, don't always put stuff in dishwasher.
- Herbicides.
- Pesticides.

What is the gut lining?

The gut lining is fragile. The gut lining is just a single layer of cells. Colon lining cells are called enterocytes.

The "front end" of enterocytes is in contact with our gut.

The "back end" of enterocytes is in contact with our immune system. The gut immune system is called GALT. Gut Associated Lymphatic Tissue.

Does leaky gut cause inflammation?

Yes. Leaky gut leads to increased bacterial endotoxin in the blood. Bacterial endotoxin is called LPS (Lipo Poly Saccharide). LPS is normally part of the cell wall of gram negative bacteria.

During digestion, proteolytic enzymes from the pancreas are secreted into the gut. These proteolytic and other enzymes cause some of the bacteria in meat, and in the colon to die.

When the gram negative bacteria die, their LPS is released into the bowel contents (succus entericus). Normally, we poop out the LPS, and it's no big deal. But if there is leaky gut, and the LPS gets beyond the enterocytes, that's a big deal.

Meat associated LPS entry into the blood is sometimes called "metabolic toxemia." The body detects the entry of LPS, and interprets it as a bacterial invasion; so an immune response is made; and the immune response causes inflammation.

LPS can bind the Toll Like Receptor, and this activates an inflammatory cascade.

What else does LPS do?

LPS can lead to increased tendency of blood to clot; That's bad.

LPS in the blood is associated with a decrease in the brain's ability to monitor, and regulate blood glucose level; this is called central insulin resistance.

What about LPS and neurodegeneration?

Douglas Kell claims that his research suggests that LPS makes fibrinogen extra coaguable, and this leads to precipitation of beta amyloid protein in the brain into insoluble aggregates.

The bigger the molecule, the more likely it is insoluble. When beta amyloid becomes insoluble, it is very difficult to remove, if not impossible.

The beta amyloid protein is a normal protein in it's original predominantly alpha helix shape.

When beta amyloid changes from it's normal alpha helix to the pleated sheet configuration, it becomes "flat."

When beta amyloid molecules are "flat," they can stack up, one on top of another, to form large insoluble aggregates.

These large insoluble aggregates can impinge on the beta amyloid alpha helices related to other cells, and cause these to convert to beta pleated sheets.

This is the mechanism of spread for a prion protein in the extracellular matrix; this is how a prion can spread from one neuronal region to another.

Note that the normal beta amyloid protein in alpha helix shape, has the SAME amino acid sequence as the abnormal prion form in pleated sheet shape.

What other ways does meat potentially cause inflammation?

Animal foods contain an acid called Neu5GC. Neu5Gc can be absorbed from the gut into the human body.

Once absorbed, it can be incorporated into human glycoproteins.

Although incorporated into human glycoproteins, Neu5Gc can still sometimes be sensed as a foreign invasion by the immune system; and provoke an autoimmune response with autoantibodies.

Meat appears to change colon bacteria to more pathogenic bacteria. Meat might lead to more Proteus bacteria. More Proteus bacteria may predispose to UTI (Urinary Tract Infection). Proteus UTI might lead to molecular mimicry with cross reactivity, and this lead to autoimmune disease like rheumatoid arthritis.

What are the common autoimmune diseases?

- Addison's disease (hypoadrenalism), alopecia areata, alopecia universalis, ankylosing spondylitis, Crohn's disease, dermatomyositis, diabetes type 1 (DM), Graves hyperthyroid, Hashimotos thyroiditis, Lupus (SLE), multiple sclerosis (MS), pernicious anemia, polymyositis, psoriasis, reiter's syndrome, relapsing polychondritis, rheumatoid arthritis (RA), scleroderma, Sjogren's syndrome, ulcerative colitis, vitiligo.

- Pitfalls include vitamin B12 deficiency is sometimes misdiagnosed as MS.

Who is Roy Swank MD?

- Roy Swank MD followed over 5,000 MS patients for decades, some for over 50 years.

- Dr Swank put MS patients on a low fat, plant based diet, and had relatively good results, with 95% of his MS patients maintaining the ability to be physically active after 34 years — unlike so many MS patients who end up severely debilitated.

- Low fat, plant diet is also associated with a lower bmi. Obese patients have increased risk of MS.

- Increased dietary sodium is associated with worse outcomes in multiple sclerosis.

What is the epidemiology of autoimmune diseases?

- More common in women, possibly related to estrogen and EDC's.
- More common in Northern areas.
- More common with obesity, which is of course associated with a meat and oil diet.

Why more in Northern areas?

- Less sunshine, and therefore less vitamin D.
- Less sunshine associated with less fruit intake.
- Possibly because more milk intake,
    - and therefore more dietary calcium,
    - and suppression of vitamin D activation,
    - from 25 hydroxy vitamin D to 1,25 hydroxy vitamin D.
- Apparently because Northerners eat more meat.

What is the benefit of ACTIVATED vitamin D = 1, 25 hydroxy vitamin D?

- Activated vitamin D regulates T cell immunity, and makes it less likely to cause autoimmune disease.

What's all that stuff about "probiotics"?

PREbiotics = fiber = food for your good gut bacteria.

PRObiotics = good gut bacteria.

POSTbiotics = the chemicals made by good gut bacteria, like butyrate.

Do I recommend taking prebiotic or probiotic supplements?

I just eat plant foods.

I don't take any supplements.

There might be a role for supplements in special situations like for treatment of antibiotic diarrhea, but I don't know.

What about fecal transplants?

Eat sh_t used to just be a metaphor.

There is a whole literature on this subject.

According to "experts," boring, wallflower, fat mice, can respond to a fecal transplant, and become skinny, swinging rockstars, like the young Elvis.

I'm skeptical.

What is recommended for most people?

Just eat a low fat, low sodium, whole food, plant diet, 100% vegan, and you will probably have a healthy gut.

Why is Parkinson's disease included as possible

autoimmune disease?

- Because the misfolded protein called alpha synuclein first shows up in the gut enteric nervous system, and this might be related to leaky gut.

- Parkinson's geographic distribution matches that of autoimmune diseases.

- Some herbicides block the metabolism of dopamine, so it's good for Parkinson's patients to only eat organic food.

- Excess iron and ROS is a big problem for Parkinson's patients. Eating 100% plant based is a way to lower iron levels.

- Vagotomy decreases the incidence of Parkinson's disease.

- Everything that happens in Vegas, stays in Vegas; but everything that happens in the gut, gets transmitted by the Vagus nerve to the brain.

What about gluten?

The protein Gluten is associated especially with wheat, rye, and barley.

This is a big topic, and entire books are written on it.

What about the diversity of our gut flora?

The more different type of plants you eat, the more different types of gut bacteria you will have.

The flexibility of our brains enables us to adapt to a wide variety of environments.

The variety of our gut bacteria enables us to eat a wide variety of foods.

What about leaky gums?

If you've got gum disease in your mouth, then oral bacteria may cause inflammation.

The best way to protect your teeth and gums is the same: 100% plant based, low fat vegan diet.

Avoid sweets.

Avoid acidic drinks like orange juice and soda pop.

At the end of the meal, rinse your mouth off with water.

When possible, clean your teeth with interdental brushes.

In the evening, you should ALWAYS floss, because at night our saliva production decreases. Never go to bed with sugar or acid in your mouth or particles of food in between your teeth.

Avoid dental trauma.

Chapter 15

Vitamin B12

Long term 100% vegans usually need to supplement with vitamin B12.

Big whoop.

B12 is usually the ONLY supplement that vegans need to take.

B12 is the only molecule in our body that contains cobalt.

What is the purpose of B12?

1. B12 is needed for some **methylation reactions**, including to make thymine for DNA, and to regulate DNA.

- Without B12, you can't make DNA correctly; instead, uracil gets inserted, and this can cause mutations in DNA.

- Inability to make thymine, is clinically indicated by abnormally large red blood cells called macrocytosis.

- The diagnostic pitfall is that a person with high folate intake might not have macrocytosis, but still be deficient in B12.

2. B12 is also needed **to convert homocysteine back into methionine**, as part of the "activated methyl cycle."

- Without B12, homocysteine accumulates.

- Homocysteine is associated with hypercoaguability, which increases risk of arterial occlusion.

- Arterial occlusion means myocardial infarction and stroke.

3. B12 is needed for **synthesis of myelin**, which is the lipid for

"insulating" neurons.

- Neurons need a normal myelin sheath for them to conduct electrical impulses correctly.

- When B12 is deficient, the myelin is made incorrectly. Incorrect myelin leads to incorrect neuronal signals.

- Incorrect neuron function can lead physical symptoms like "pins and needles," or psychiatric symptoms like moodiness, depression, and cognitive impairment.

What about folate?

- Folate is dependent on B12 for regeneration of the active form of Folate. Folate deficiency also causes inability to make thymine for DNA.

- Folate comes from "Foliage," also known as plants. Folia in Latin means "leaf." Greens and beans are excellent sources of folate.

- **FOLATE** helps prevent cancer, by maintaining Thymine levels.

- If folate is deficient, then thymine levels drop, and uracil gets inserted into DNA. **Uracil insertion into DNA causes mutations**.

- Folate is a methyl donor. Some folate donated methyl groups are used for histone and DNA methylation. Abnormal DNA methylation can potentially activate oncogenes and promote cancer.

- In the chapter on vitamin C, we talked about vitamin C helping to regulate DNA synthesis.

- These are just two examples, folate and vitamin C, of plant supplied nutrients that decrease risk of cancer.

- Tap water often contains chemicals that inhibit the activity of folate. Eating plant foods, provides high amounts of folate, and vitamin C, to overcome this inhibition of folate.

- Tea can contain chemicals that inhibit the activity of folate. Tea also tends to concentrate aluminum. This combination of lowered folate activity, and increased aluminum, can decrease cognitive function. I recommend to avoid drinking tea, and to filter your drinking water with reverse osmosis.

What's the key point about the chemistry of folate and B12?

They are METHYL DONORS in "methyl cycle." This one carbon metabolism-methyl cycle is essential for DNA synthesis, and regulation of DNA synthesis.

Folate and B12 are dependent on each other in the "methyl cycle."

If a cell can't make DNA correctly, it usually either 1. dies, or 2. functions poorly, or 3. becomes cancerous.

Folate deficiency is associated with increased risk of colon cancer and some other cancers.

What diseases have signs and symptoms that overlap with B12 deficiency?

Folate deficiency is associated with macrocytosis.

Multiple sclerosis, Bell's palsy, fibromyalgia, chronic fatigue syndrome, change in behavior, depression, Lyme disease, and tertiary Syphilis, limbic encephalitis, can have neurologic symptoms that overlap with B12 deficiency.

It is wise to always check for B12 deficiency, because it is so easy to treat.

How does B12 present in children?

All of the above, and-or behavior problems, and learning disability.

What does that mean in plain English?

If your wife or kid is acting crazier than usual, then check a B12 blood level.

What diseases can occur in association with B12 deficiency?

B12 deficiency in 100% vegans is a DIETARY deficiency, and therefore an isolated problem.

B12 deficiency can be due to an autoimmune disease. Autoimmune diseases often come in groups of two or three.

Therefore, if B12 deficiency seems due to autoimmune disease like pernicious anemia, one should check for other autoimmune diseases like Hashimoto's, Grave's, or Addison's; and one should avoid things that cause leaky gut.

Where does B12 come from?

B12 is made by bacteria. DNA is not made by plants or animals.

B12 is in the dirt, but we usually remove the dirt from our food; and we peel our carrots.

We tend to peel many other foods including potatos.

Nowadays, so much herbicides and pesticides are put on crops, that not that much B12 comes from the soil.

Eating animal foods does provide B12.

I think it is better to obtain B12 from oral supplements.

What are the steps for B12 absorption from food?

In your mouth, B12 binds to haptocorrin, which protects it from stomach acid.

In your duodenum, B12 binds to intrinsic factor.

In your ileum, the B12 is absorbed into the blood.

Where is extra B12 stored?

In the liver.

What is a normal B12 level?

In general, 200 pg/ml is often given as a threshold for a normal B12 level.

However, some experts recommend using 350 pg/ml as a threshold for normal.

Different laboratories have slightly different ranges for defining a "normal" B12 level.

The last time I checked my B12 level, the lab company defined "normal" as 230-1300 pg/ml.

I think 230 is too low.

I only take B12 once a month, so I like to have a "safety reserve" above the 350 threshold that is recommended by experts.

I like to keep my B12 at least 500. **between 500-1,500 pg/ml**.

I take 5,000 micrograms of **sublingual, methylcobalamin** B12, **once a month**. That's it.

Some B12 experts recommend a daily dose or a weekly dose.

I find it more convenient to just take it once a month.

I have checked my blood levels, and I know this works well for me.

Can a person have a "normal" blood level, but still be

deficient in B12?

Yes, but that is uncommon.
For example, a person could have depleted bodily stores of B12, but they might have just took a sublingual tablet before the blood draw, resulting in a "normal" blood level.

Sometimes the lab has an error in measurement.

Some persons require blood levels of over 350 for optimal neuronal function.

Why is B12 deficiency much more common in females?

I don't know, but it might be because monthly menstruation.   Need extra B12 to make all those RBC's every month.

Why are women called "Fe-males"?

Because you have to pay a lot of "fees" if you want a woman to stay with you; or if one divorces you.

When else might a person need some extra B12?

Wound healing.

Pregnancy.

What can be done if the doctor thinks the patient is B12 deficient despite a "normal" blood level?

The doctor can check blood levels of Methyl Malonic Acid (MMA). MMA is elevated with B12 deficiency. An elevated MMA level helps show that the problem is due to a lack of B12, and not due folate deficiency.

Distinction between folate and B12 arises, because either one can cause macrocytosis; and macrocytosis is often the first thing noticed on a complete blood count (CBC), which is a commonly ordered blood test.

Macrocytosis and elevated homocysteine can both occur from a folate deficiency.

If B12 level is borderline, and homocysteine is high, then the elevated homocysteine might lead your doctor to consider B12 supplementation..

The doctor might recommend supplementing with B12 for a few months, to see if symptoms improve.

What's the best way to take B12?

I avoid cy--ano-cobalamin. I don't want to eat anything with the word "cy--ano" in it.

There are hydroxyl and methyl forms of cobalamin.
Methylcobalamin is photosensitive, so the container needs to be opaque.

I prefer methylcobalamin sublingual. The fewer the ingredients the better.

Methylcobalamin is the active form in our body.

By taking a sublingual B12, you avoid all the problems of intestinal B12 absorption.

If a person has digestive problems with their stomach or small bowel, they might not be able to absorb B12.

These persons might be able to maintain normal blood levels of B12 by taking sublingual B12, or by B12 injections.

Hydroxycobalamin is the form often used for injections.

Who does B12 injections?

Doctors perform B12 injections.

Why use injections when B12 can be given

sublingually or orally?

Some people have decreased function of their intestinal tract, and can't absorb B12.

For acutely symptomatic, B12 deficient persons, it's good to try to raise blood levels quickly; before neurologic symptoms become irreversible.

B12 injections are the fastest, most reliable way to increase B12 levels.

For a heathly vegan, sublingual B12 is sufficient.

I have never had a B12 injection, and I doubt that I will ever need one.

How do you know if your B12 dose is correct?

Check your B12 blood levels.

About Author

PR fits no category; he's the preCambrian, rabbit fossil of nutrition writers.

He became famous for discovering that the archeopteryx "fossil" is just a photograph of a fruit fly smooshed on the wall in the shower stall.

PR is the founder of:[20]

- Meat eaters anonymous.

- End nutritional ignorance foundation.

- Puerto Rican doctors for world domination (a group who intend to take over the world, and make everyone learn Spanish, and conjugate verbs in the subjunctive).

- AC-LOG-WTTM[21]

How his wife sees him: a disturbingly amorous robot, who makes money for her.

How his kids see him: a waste of life, who dresses like a bum, and sits around the house, reading all the time.

How he sees himself: a nutrition scholar — like the scholastics Albert the Dominican, and Thomas Aquinas,[22]

or the humanists, like Petrarch and Ficino[23] — maintaining the medical and

---

20 Just joking.

21 American College —of Lonely Old Guys — Who Talk Too Much

22 **Albert** the Dominican wrote the commentaries on Aristotle that established scholasticism. **Aquinas** refined the ideas of Aristotle to the zenith of scholasticism, that doubled the IQ of the middle ages.

23 **Petrarch** discovered the letters of Cicero, that began the Italian renaissance. **Ficino**, physician-philosopher, devoted his life to translating the works of Plato, and other Greeks, which guided the Italians to a new apex of art, like Raphael's "School of Athens."

nutritional knowledge of the past, for the future renaissance in health.

Ficino burned candles to a bust of Plato.

"Aristotle's genius is purely human, but Plato's is both human and divine."
- Marsilio Ficino.

I prefer Aristotle over Plato, but I admire Ficino's enthusiasm.

Enthusiasm is a prerequisite for great achievement.

Great ages like Periclean Athens, Raphaelen Rome, and Victorian England, are characterized by high wealth, high art, **an energizing myth**, and awesome architecture.

Athens had the Parthenon. Ancient Rome had the Pantheon. Renaissance Rome had Michelangelo's basilica. England had Wren's, and Pugin's cathedrals.

And what great architecture ennobles us?

"Modern corporate buildings look like animal cages, and they all have a statue of a turd in front."
- Tom Wolfe.

How inspiring.

What art can inspire us?

Athens had Phidias. The renaissance had the above. The counter reformation had Caravaggio. Victorian England had the Pre-Raphaelite brotherhood.

What art does the modern world have?

I'm not aware of any great art since Norman Rockwell, Roberto Innocenti, Arnold Friberg, Don Troiani, Bev Doolittle, and Robert Bateman.

I would like to commission a new painting for the nutritional renaissance. The painting will be based on Raphael's "School of Athens."

It will be called, "**School of Veganism**."

John McDougall will take the place of Plato in the center, pointing upward with a potato to represent starch.

Dennis Burkitt will stand next to him, taking the place of Aristotle, and pointing to the ground to remind us of fiber, and its effects.

Then the other great nutrition experts — like T. Colin Campbell, Caldwell Esselstyn, Walter Kempner, Peter Cleave, Hugh Trowell, Dean Ornish, Nathan Pritikin, Ancel Keys, Michael Greger, Cyrus Wombatta, Bobby Bigpoo, Chef AJ, Rich Roll, and others — will be positioned on both sides, with their groups of students around them. I will take the place of Diogenes, looking like a homeless person, alone, seated on the steps.

Starch, fruits and vegetables will be the new "Trivium" of nutrition education.

Perhaps we should pattern the school after Plato's Academy, and call it "Nutricademy."

Or perhaps after Aristotle's Lyceum, it could be called "Nutrium."

Other than a lack of funds, or education, or interest: a nutritional renaissance is just around the corner.

Where are the Medici's when you need them?[24]

"Eloquence without finance finds no ears."   - anonymous.

"Renaissance scholars taught man to celebrate life, rather than brood about death… renaissance artists put paganism into Christian art, and made it better."

                                                        - Will Durant.

How my high school daughter explains my lack of book sales?

She was shown a column I wrote in 7th grade for the local, recreation center, comedy newsletter.

She said, "You haven't matured at all since 7th grade. Your writing has the same stupid jokes and misplaced metaphors."

---

24 The **Medici** family were the greatest patrons of art in the history of the world. They supported Ficino, Botticelli, and Michelangelo.

How does the wife explain my lack of book sales?

"The reason no one reads your books is because you talk about yourself too much."   - Wife.

As if leaving out this little "about the author" section would make any difference.

She just wants me to quit this penniless habit; and start moonlighting; to make more money, that she can steal.

She doesn't know that I'm going to retire soon, and then mooch off of *HER*. Ha, ha!

How is this book different from the others?

Now, in the late 50's, the author has outgrown the adolescent silliness of his early 50's.

Comparison with other artists?

During his whole life, Vincent van Gogh only sold one painting.

I sold two books to my cousin (who bought them out of pity). So I'm ahead of van Gogh.

How can the readers be sure that this book is not corporate sponsored?

What readers? This book has no publisher, no testimonials, no advertising, and no sales. How much more authentic can it be?

Why should anyone take you seriously about nutrition?

I'm 57, but I read at the 58 year old level.

I'm not the guy to ask about getting laid, or getting paid, but I do know a lot about medical stuff.

In the first year of medical school, I believed that the key to becoming a great doctor would be to understand biochemistry, because that was the language of God, to write the book of life.

In medical school, I got 780 out of 800 on biochemistry boards, which is around 99.99 percentile, maybe the highest in the country.

A bunch of other similar academic achievements.

When a doctor looks at a brain MRI, or CT angiogram, of course, the goal is to accurately describe the findings.

Then one can ask, "Why did this brain shrink, stroke, or bleed?"

I notice that the same patients with amyloid angiopathy, often have hypertensive retinopathy, and diabetic retinopathy.

Studying what causes hypertension and diabetes, leads to papers on sodium, fructose, lipids, and atherosclerosis.

Most disease is caused by bad diet and toxic exposures; to understand disease one has to read about nutrition, and estrogenic chemicals.

To me the "standard" is just a beginning.

Do retarded people deserve the standard of care? Of course they do.

Do demented people deserve the standard of care? Of course they do.

Do intoxicated people deserve the standard of care? Of course they do.

Do unconscious people deserve the standard of care? Of course they do.

The standard of care is for retarded, demented, intoxicated, unconscious people; the standard requires no effort from the patient.

An intelligent, motivated person should want more than the standard. Standard implies average. Average is synonymous with obese and unhealthy.

A literate person should want **OPTIMAL** health.

I have been on a quest for decades to understand OPTIMAL health, and OPTIMAL cognitive performance.

Most people think that science just keeps on progressing, and that the textbooks are getting better and better.

That is not true. The "standard" textbooks for chronic diseases are out of date. People are getting fatter and sicker.

Academic, attending physicians do not get promoted for writing textbooks, so they assign the task to junior fellows who don't know anything; and the junior fellows just copy the old edition, and many textbooks are 50-100 years out of date.

There is a big gap between the scientific literature, and the standard textbooks.

This gap energized me to plow through countless articles, and books of biochemistry, nutrition, pathophysiology, radiology, history, philosophy, etc.

I could easily teach at least half the freshman & sophomore classes offered at any university.

I routinely zoom through college dvd and medical CME (continuing medical education) courses in multiple fields at 2.5x speed.

Like Aeneas, who carried his father, Anchises, out of burning Troy, I carry my father in my head.

I'm from a Trojan too.[25]

Aeneas went on to have an affair with the beautiful, Carthaginian, princess Dido.

Where's my princess Dido?

My wife would say, "You want a Dido? Just add an "L" to her name, and shove it!"

My wife was sad about one of her friends having an unhappy marriage. Trying to cheer her up, I said, "Well, at least I've never cheated on you."

Wife: That doesn't count.

Me: Whaddya mean?

Wife: No one wants you. You're short, bald, ugly, and autistic!

Me: You're just jealous, because I'm aging better than you!

Mirror, mirror, on the wall, who is aging best of all?

The Alfred Adler inferiority principle shows that a weakness, can motivate a strength.

Michelangelo felt unattractive, because of his broken nose, so he avoided social situations. Rumor has it that Michelangelo was a virgin. He

_____

25 With a hole in it.

compensated by putting more time into his art.

I compensate for my social limitations by putting more time into studying nutrition and health.

Freud would describe this as sublimating one's romantic impulses into creative work.

Yeah sure, every guy dreams of being a King with a harem, or at least a hot wife, that drives like a sports car, but almost all guys end up with a mini-van, and then the majority get divorced.

You've come a long way baby?

In hunter gatherer groups, a woman breast feeds her baby for at least 3 years, and has 10 or more kids. She is with her children all day.

In Victorian England, a woman was expected to be a virgin before marriage, and would then typically have 10-15 kids, and she did not work outside the home.

The modern woman is more academically educated than the hunter gatherer, or Victorian woman, but is she *biologically* smarter?

Nowadays, a woman has often slept with 10 men before marriage, and often has a venereal disease.

She then has 2 kids, often by C-section (so have limited gut bacteria); breast feeds for 3 months or less; feeds them unfiltered water, and microwaved, BPA bottle, formula milk which lowers IQ;

then she is away from them almost all day, because she has a job;

then she divorces the husband, so kid grows up without a male role model, and no parent in the house;

then sends kid to a school that teaches him that life is meaningless, and the only reason to study, or work, is for money.

Then her "maternal" instincts make her buy dogs, who she talks to as if they were her children.

Being an empty nest, dog lady is better than being a spinster, cat lady; but it's usually happier to have a family with kids home for the holidays, papa, grandma and grandpa at her side.

In her dreams.

What progress civilization has made.

No wonder modern society has become idiocracy.

"The best a man can do is to learn about the good things in civilization and try to transmit this to the next generation...

Civilizations begin with religion and stoicism:

they end with... unbelief, and the undisciplined pursuit of individual pleasure.

A civilization is born stoic and dies epicurean."   - Will Durant.

The end of belief is the end of art.

Why strive to create art, if life has no meaning?

Atheism doesn't know the difference between art and a fart.

There's more to life than social media.

For the few, who enjoy learning for its own sake, their reading becomes an enduring pleasure.

Our fate should be something better than to become a bunch of illiterate, fatsos.

"The habit of learning is the greatest pleasure, because it can be enjoyed continuously for hours; unlike the other pleasures which quickly wax and wane."   - Aristotle.

"That I can read and be happy while I am reading, is a great blessing.
This habit of reading... is your pass to the greatest, the purest, and most perfect pleasure that God has prepared for his creatures.
It lasts when all other pleasures fade... It will make your hours pleasant as long as you live."   - Anthony Trollope.

"Everything takes longer than it should, except sex."   - anonymous.

Aeneas went on to found Rome.

I have no where to go.

Like Newton, alone in the country, hiding from the plague, with only his books, before "anno mirabilis," when he enlightened the world with discoveries in optics, mechanics, and calculus.

No, really. Why do you write nutrition books?

What else am I gonna do?

If I moonlight for money, my wife will see the opportunity for a big alimony check — like a shark senses blood in the water — and divorce me.

My wife is about as interested in me as Daphne was in Apollo.[26]

I don't have enough money to attract a mistress. When a man is as ugly as me, mistresses don't come cheap.

"I don't avoid temptation. Temptation avoids me."   - anonymous.

Why don't I travel with the family?

Yeah, right. Agoraphobia prevents me from going anywhere.

The family goes on vacation for ten days, and here's the return conversation.

Daughter: Dad, you must have been lonely with no one around to check their reflection on your head.

Me: Nice, double insult; Short and bald.

Daughter: Dad, you really should buy some new clothes. You look like a homeless person. You look like St Francis of Assisi after methampheetamine.

Why not socialize with friends?

Assburger syndrome prevents developing friendships, so weekends are just a time for more reading.

Like a koala bear foraging for eucalyptus leaves, I forage for knowledge leafing through books.

Who is the best doctor?

The one who can save the most patients.

---

26 "Daphne and Apollo," statue by Lorenzo Bernini, 1622.

Who is the doctor that can save the most patients?

The doctor who best understands the causes of disease.

Why is understanding causation so important?

The best way to cure a disease is to remove the cause.

When a doctor tells you that he doesn't know what causes your disease, what he is really saying is that he doesn't know how to cure your disease.

Which doctor best understands the causes of diseases?

The doctor who best understands nutrition, and pathophysiology.

I know that I'm on to something with the study of nutrition, and pathophysiology.

Most doctors only know their own field. The big name university centers are chasing grant money, not understanding.

I trained at Harvard and other big name places. I know what they know.

When I was at Harvard, the vascular surgeons hated the interventional radiologists, because they felt that IR was taking their cases. Cardiologists had contempt for IR, because they believed that IR was clinically incompetent.

We had a weekly conference with PV surgery and cardiology. No one from IR wanted to present cases, because they would mock us.

I saw it as an opportunity, and volunteered to present every week. I read the surgery journals, and the cardiology journals. I watched the surgery and cardiology VHS courses. I did elective rotations in their specialties. I know what they know.
Vascular surgeons care about surgery, not pathophysiology. Cardiologists care about stents, not pathophysiology. Internists care about pharmacology, not pathophysiology.

One of the big surprises is that knowledge often comes from unexpected places. The best experts on diabetes, are not diabetes doctors. The best experts are type one diabetics themselves who have studied their disease as if their life depended on it, because it does.

The best expert on vitamin B12 is not an endocrinologist or neurologist or hematologist from a big name place; it's a general practitioner, Dr Chandy, who studied B12 so he could help his daughter, and then realized he could help a lot of patients.

Alexander the Great slept with a copy of the "Iliad" under his pillow, and dreamed that he might be the next Achilles.

I sleep with a copy of Burkitt's biography under my pillow, and dream that I might be the next, great synthesizer of pathophysiology patterns; someone who can see the connections between the different fields.

Great experts can't be from a research hospital, because there is too much pressure to focus on reductionist topics to obtain grant money.

Great experts can't be specialists, because specialists are too caught up in the details of their own field. A cardiologist cannot criticize stents. A vascular surgeon cannot criticize open, arterial, bypass surgery.

It has to be a genralist who understands the connections between biochemistry, nutrition, pathology, surgery, and radiology. Someone who can recognize the brilliance of Douglas Kell PhD, but also see that he's over his head, because he's fat.

Anyone who understands nutrition is not fat. To be fat is a public announcement that you don't understand nutrition, and pathophysiology.

Why shouldn't I become one of the best experts in the world for understanding chronic disease?

Yeah sure, McDougall, Barnard, and Ornish have more direct patient care experience than me. Campbell has a more lab research than me. Sloop has more pathology knowledge than me.

But I've got a lot more experience than all of them put together for looking at patterns of chronic disease on ultrasound, DSA, CT, CTA, PET, MRI, and MRA, and correlating these with nutrition, and pathophysiology.

This is the most valuable knowledge in the world, but there's no money in it, because companies can't profit from it, and the patient's are too ignorant to seek it.

Most doctors think chronic disease is hopeless: the only thing that can be done is to try to slow it down, a little bit, with medications.

Every week I solve several complex, brain, neck, and spine cases based on reading outside my main fields.

To be competent, a doctor has to read in their own field.

To excel, a doctor has to read in multiple other fields.

When I was a 3rd year medical student on the wards, the residents mocked biochemistry saying, "What ya learned about "glycolysis" ain't gonna help ya on the wards, for taking care of patients."

I figured they were right, and ignored biochem for 20 years. But then I returned to it, because it's the best way to explain the mechanisms of many diseases.

Once you know what causes a disease, you can teach the patient to avoid it.

Sadly, it's very rare that patients with chronic disease ever improve. They almost always progressively deteriorate.

I used to think chronic disease was depressing. Every morning **RIVERS** of fat, diabetics flow into hospitals.

After studying chronic disease for a thirty years, I realized that chronic disease has an **Achilles heel.**

The shocking discovery is that **70% OF DISEASE IS CAUSED BY BAD DIET** and **ESTROGENICS**: meat, oils, refined sugar, food additives, and of course alcohol, and tobacco.

These can all be avoided!!!

Every day, I see a bunch of blindness, strokes, degenerated brains, and spines, and amputated feet.

Most can be **PREVENTED** by low fat, low sodium, whole food, vegan diet, and water filtration.

Much of it can even be **REVERSED** by a low fat, low sodium, vegan diet; and avoiding estrogenics, tobacco, and alcohol.

I find myself in a bizarre position. I have the knowledge of disease prevention, that could help millions of people, but they don't want to be helped, because they are too ignorant.

Human intelligence = IQ x Curiosity x objectivity.

Most people have adequate IQ's; their problem is ZERO curiosity!

IQ of 200 x Curiosity of ZERO = zero.

Other people also have plenty of IQ, and even some curiosity, but they lack objectivity. If you criticize their diet go into a Kung Fu Kata of defensive rationalizations.

Any moron can eat rice, beans, potatos, sweet potatoes, and oat meal.

However, less than 1% of persons seems able to **CHANGE** from eating the MOFU diet to eating healthy.

If you ask them to sign consent for a complex surgery, they say, "Oh sure." If you ask them to eat plant foods, they say, "No, not that!"

How could people not be fascinated by nutrition?

Nutrition is what connects anatomy, health, and disease. Nutrition is the key to understanding disease, and radiology (imaging of disease).

The main reason people are not curious, is because they think they already know enough about nutrition, and that it's not important.

Most people are sick because they are ignorant. It's not

genetic. It's not because they're getting older.

When I first realized this, I thought, "Hurray! I'm gonna save all these lives, and become rich!"

I felt like God had given me the keys to health heaven.[27]

The sick people would be in line, and I would walk past them with a sign that says "*100% vegan*," and then the lame shall walk, like in the painting, "St Peter healing with his shadow" by Masaccio.[28]

Then I learned about the Dunning Kruger effect — ignorant people don't realize they're ignorant.

- **Dunning-Kruger effect** = Incompetent people tend to overestimate their own ability, because they are too incompetent to judge it.

---

27 **"Giving the keys to St Peter"** by Perugino, painted in 1482 for Sistine chapel.
28 **"St Peter healing with his shadow"** by Masaccio, painted in 1420 for the Brancacci chapel.

- Like a teenager who thinks they know more than their parents.

You can lead a horse to water, but you can't make him drink.
You can send a kid to college, but you can't make him think.
You can show a fatso to the benefits of vegan diet, but you can't make them link.

When you correct an ignorant person, they don't say, "Thank you." They get mad at you.

"Rebuke a mocker, and he will hate you; rebuke a wise man, and he will love you."
- Proverbs 9:8.

"In theory, it is easy to convince an ignorant person; in actual life, men not only object to offer themselves to be convinced, but hate the man who has convinced them."
- Epictetus.

"As a dog returneth to his vomit, so a fool returneth to his folly."

- Proverbs 26:11.

"Talk sense to a fool, and he calls you foolish."   - Euripides.

"It is difficult to free fools from the chains they love."   - Voltaire.

If you talk to the typical person they will say, "I'm not illiterate."

Then ask them, "What books did you read this month?

They will say, "Uhh. I've been real busy."

Then ask them, "What books did you read this year?"

Same answer.

Not wanting to read, has the same effect as not being able to read.

I think to myself, "I'm sorry that they made you read Caesar salad, Great Expectorations, Micklberry Finn, and Seduce a Mockingbird when you were a freshman in high school. And you became convinced that "reading" was a painful, waste of time; but that doesn't give you the right to never read another book in your life."

God gave us a brain so that we could learn, and think.

Our skill with language is the main thing that separates us from animals.

"The ordinary person, especially in the villages, knows absolutely nothing... they live like simple cattle." - Martin Luther.

I decided to build a Gothic cathedral hospital devoted to VEGANISM, with painted murals explaining how to become a vegan. The carved statues would includes lots of before and after people who became skinny.

I made the design for the Gothic Hospital. Each specialty had its own statue.

The statue for diagnostic radiology is the performance of a barium enema; for cardiac surgery a circular saw on the sternum.

Even though we know that men and women are exactly the same, there was always a crowd of teenage boys staring at the statue of the gyne speculum exam, but hardly any women spent much time by the statue of the man undergoing ureteral catheterization for cystoscopy.

A lot of women did seem curious about the man undergoing a wallet biopsy.

My medical friends loved the Gothic statues, but all the patients got scared. I ended up having to sell the blueprints to one of those haunted house, wax museum places.

Given that most Americans do NOT read books — I don't think we're gonna see a bunch of skinny vegans walking around any time soon.

Is it reasonable that our average citizen has become obese and illiterate?

"Until at last, having educated himself into imbecility, and polluted, and drugged himself into stupefaction, he keeled over — a weary, battered old brontosaurus — and became extinct." - Malcolm Muggeridge.

"Consider your origins: you were not made to live as brutes, but to follow virtue and knowledge."

- Dante.

I know lots of people in the medical business, and less than 1% of them is a 100%, low fat, low sodium, whole food vegan.

Boob tube videos of low carb, BS artists are like sheep dogs, to corral the immoral majority into a downward, diagonal decline of degenerative disease.

The exit door of fast food restaurants leads to a hospital. Fast food restaurants are the best source of *referrals* for hospitals.

By 40, the average frustrated chump (AFC) has dipped his toe into the outer edge of the sickness whirlpool.

By 50, the typical AFC is spiraling downwards into health hell; the land of impotence, diabetes, heart disease, and despair.

The "good fats — everything in moderation — mediterranean diet" crowd ends up prematurely subterranean.

"Good fats" and "mediterranean diet" are just marketing slogans to make chumps think it's okay to eat meat and oils.

I do like mediterranean names with all those vowels like Orlando Enamorato, and Gino Cellini Bigpini.

Maybe I should change my name to Pierro Rogero?

Oh, why couldn't God have made me tall (women are suckers for tall guys), or rich (rich people don't have to labor for money).

Eventually, we learn to accept our fate, and to embrace it.

God has made me a nutrition nerd, and I shall live that role to the fullest.

Time for meditation. The mantra is:

"It could be worse.

 It could be worse.

   Focus on her breasts.

   Focus on..."

Other books by this author

Rhyme, rhetoric and logic.

How to fix your fat azz in five easy steps.

A tale of two toes, and a hot tub: How to improve blood flow.

Ischemic spine is most common cause of back pain.

How to reduce risk of cancer and chronic disease.

Straight A at Stanford and on to Harvard.

Wisdom quotes.

How to raise IQ and become a genius.

Vegan reformation.

Pocket radiologist interventional procedures.

Medical student's guide to top board scores.

Quick medical Spanish.

You tube channel is "**Peter Rogers MD**."

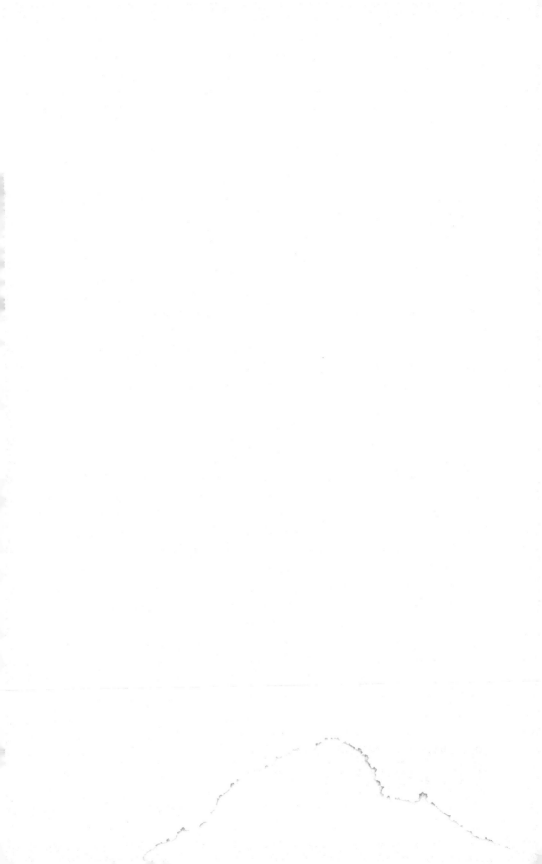

Made in the USA
Monee, IL
28 June 2021